D1084646

The Practice of
Community-Oriented Primary Health Care

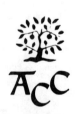

APPLETON-CENTURY-CROFTS / New York

The Practice of
Community-Oriented
Primary
Health Care

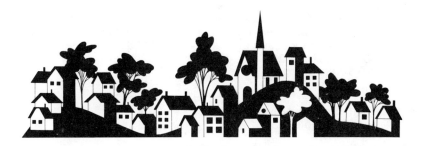

SIDNEY L. KARK, M.D.

Professor and Chairman, the Haim Yassky Department of Social
Medicine, School of Public Health and Community Medicine, The
Hebrew University-Hadassah Medical School and Hadassah–
Hebrew University Medical Center, Jerusalem, Israel

Prentice-Hall International, Inc., London
Prentice-Hall of Australia, Pty. Ltd., Sydney
Prentice-Hall of India Private Limited, New Delhi
Prentice-Hall of Japan, Inc., Tokyo
Prentice-Hall of Southeast Asia (Pte.) Ltd., Singapore
Whitehall Books Ltd., Wellington, New Zealand

Library of Congress Cataloging in Publication Data

Kark, Sidney L
  The practice of community-oriented primary
health care.

  Includes index.
  1. Community health services. I. Title.
[DNLM: 1. Community health services. 2. Community
medicine. 3. Primary health care. WA546.1 K18p]
RA425.K357   362.1′0425   80-17639
ISBN 0-8385-7865-9

Cover Design: Gloria J. Moyer
Text Design: Alan Gold

CONTENTS

PREFACE

In my book, *Epidemiology and Community Medicine,* published in 1974, one section was a consideration of the practice of community medicine and primary health care, and the possibility of bringing together medical practice in the community with health care conducted by public health agencies. Several reviewers, and other correspondents, expressed particular interest in this aspect of the book and in our endeavors toward finding new forms of community health care.

Since then, a tremendous spate of publications on primary health care is evidence of a worldwide trend toward this area of health. What was until comparatively recently a neglected aspect of health services has thus become a main focus of attention in both developed and developing countries. Evidence of this in more developed countries is the recent vitalization of family medicine in the United States, and the analogous growth in stature of the general practitioner in the United Kingdom. At the same time, community medicine has developed in these countries. In my view, it is an important area of the older and broader field of public health, a discipline which extends beyond community medicine and personal health care to the environmental sciences and engineering.

There has been an unfortunate separation between community medicine and primary health care. Although community medicine is concerned with the health of the community as a whole, there is no reason why primary health care should be confined to the treatment and care of individual patients. In fact, there is a strong case for enlarging the traditional horizons of the primary care practitioner from the strictly clinical to the epidemiologic and community aspects of care. It is this which I refer to as community-oriented primary health care.

The chapters in this book focus on several facets of community-oriented primary health care. The first three chapters review the subjects of community health care; community diagnosis and health surveillance in primary health care; and the health team for such care. The principles and practices of community-oriented primary health care have universal relevance. Two chapters, 4 and 8, review the development of such practices in the contrasting settings of a city neighborhood and a rural peasant community. Illustrations of its application to different age groups, and to the identified problems of different communities, are presented in Chapters 5, 6, and 7 in an urban community, and in Chapter 9 in a rural peasant community.

This book is directed toward those who are interested in the development of primary health care as a practice that not only responds to the expressed needs of individual patients seeking care and treatment when ill, but also functions with communities and families as a public health or community medicine practice in promoting community health.

There have been many pilot projects in community health in Africa, the Americas, Asia, and Europe, but the countrywide establishment of a network of health care units as part of social policy is a comparatively recent phenomenon. This can no longer depend on the personality and drive of innovative leaders, but demands careful planning of manpower needs and training. For this purpose, existing and new pilot projects should be developed as field training areas (FTAs); and schools of medicine, nursing, and public health should be encouraged to incorporate such FTAs as an integral part of their programs. Surely, the FTA is as essential for training health professionals and auxiliaries in community health care as are the wards of a hospital for training in hospital medicine and nursing.

Unless this fresh approach to community health and medical care is attempted, personal health services will make little contribution to improving the health of communities. Changes in the environment and socioeconomic progress are the main factors recognized as having produced advances in the health status of communities. It is our belief, borne out by experience in different settings, that even where the social climate is not promising, the approach of community-oriented primary health care can do much to improve people's health. The health professions need a modified motivation, orientation, and training to do this. The need for active involvement and research in this direction is an urgent challenge to schools of public health, medical and nursing schools, and national health institutes.

ACKNOWLEDGMENTS

I continue to be indebted to many colleagues, past and present, for the stimulating life experience it has been my good fortune to share with them in applying basic epidemiologic, social, and public health precepts in the development of community-oriented primary health care.

My wife, Dr. Emily Kark, has been closely identified and professionally involved in whatever principles and practices of community-oriented primary health care we have developed over the past 40 years. She has helped in critical review and editing of the entire book, and is a joint author of Chapters 8 and 9.

I would especially like to pay tribute, and express my deep gratitude, to the founder members of the team responsible for our early development of community-oriented primary health care in the rural community of Polela. Associated with my wife and myself were Edward Jali (medical aide), his wife, Amelia Jali (the first state registered nurse at Polela), and the original group of community health workers, who had previously been malaria control workers in other parts of the country. Very shortly after the project's initiation, Polela men and women were invited to join the staff of the health center and were trained as community health workers. Outstanding among them were Margaret Nzimande-Shembe, Audrey and Ernest Bennie, Benjamin Nzimande, Fred Madlala, and Raphael Zaca.

The experiences with community health care in a city neighborhood, which are analyzed in several chapters, are continuing in the Hadassah community health center, Kiryat Yovel, Jerusalem. It is rare that an organization of a developed country should initiate and maintain, in a less developed country, a program of health care that is not a replica or product of its own country's health service system. It is just this that has been done in Kiryat Yovel by the Hadassah Medical Organization. To the organization itself, and especially to Dr. K. J. Mann, its Director-General in Israel, I would like to pay tribute and to thank them for their continuing support of our new approaches to community health care. This center has become the field training area, not only for nursing and medical students, but for graduate students in public health. In it, the partnership between the Hebrew University and Hadassah is pioneering new avenues of graduate education in public health and community medicine.

Over a number of years, we have developed field workshops in community-oriented primary health care, in which the potential public health significance of different primary care practices is studied. I am especially grateful to our graduate students in public health, and our medical residents, for their critical observations and studies of our approach. They have made a number of important contributions to our practice and to development of theory.

An important feature of the community health center in Jerusalem has been the close association of the health center team and others in the university department of social medicine. Together they have developed the various community medicine programs in the framework of the neighborhood primary care services provided by the center. It is impossible to name all those who have been involved in this process and to whom I am deeply indebted. The key members are:

Epidemiology and Biostatistics: J. H. Abramson, E. Peritz, H. Palti, E. Simchen, J. Gofin, R. Gofin, I. Ronen, B. Adler, and M. Avizur. Dr H. Palti is the joint author of Chapter 5.

Community Health Care:
Family Health and Home Care: B. Gampel, C. Hopp, R. Bah
Maternal and Child Health: Z. Shamir, H. Palti, D. Flug, M. Gitlin, I. Belmaker
Family and Community Nursing: H. Derenberg-Kurtzman, P. Karpf, R. Elishkovsky, G. Helman, H. Kossovsky, B. Lis, Y. Moskowitz, S. Weiner, D. Block, and R. Pogrond.
Others: R. Cohen (Laboratory), L. Weinbach (Pharmacy), M. Zur (Administration).

Health Behavior: H. Pridan, I. Cohen, N. Mainemer.

Community Mental Health: I. Levav.

I would also like to express my appreciation to my colleagues in the medical school and Hadassah for their support.

Finally, I would like to thank Mrs. B. Slonim, departmental administrator, and her secretarial staff, for their invaluable assistance and typing of the manuscript for this book.

The Practice of
Community-Oriented Primary Health Care

CHAPTER 1

COMMUNITY HEALTH CARE

Health care is provided to communities by a variety of discrete and often independently functioning health services. Some of these services are located in the community to which they deliver care, while others are not. The health of a community in an urban neighborhood or rural village may be considerably influenced by public health and hospital services that are not necessarily located in it or focused specifically on it. They contribute to the health of such local communities as part of their more widely distributed programs. Most of the major advances in the provision of health care have been by hospital and public health services rather than by services that are focused on and based in the local community itself. These will be considered before going on to more detailed consideration of community health care.

HOSPITAL CARE

A tremendous investment has been and continues to be made in the development of hospitals, with the result that a great part of total expenditure on health care is spent on these institutions and a major proportion of the health professions work in hospitals. In the United Kingdom, the initial spending on hospitals was estimated to be 55 percent of the total expenditure of the National Health Service, rising to over 65 percent in the first 25 years of the service.[1] This increase is reflected in the proportion of personnel employed in hospital services—over nine times as much as in community services.

The best-equipped hospitals are those for acute or short-stay cases rather than those for the long-term patient who is mentally or physically disabled. They reach their greatest technologic development as teaching and research hospitals, in which treatment of the individual patient has reached a standard of technical excellence that has made these institutions preeminent in clinical research and teaching. The modern multidepartmental hospital is the major field of clinical practice for undergraduate and postgraduate students in medicine and nursing, and has been so in the Western world for a considerable time. Thus, it is regarded as the center of health care by the medical professions and the public. The growth of a wide array of specialities of clinical medicine has taken place in the hospital, with the result that it is composed of many departments, each with its beds for inpatients, its clinics, its special equipment, and often its own laboratories. Each has right of access to central facilities of the hospital, which themselves consist of specialty units, such as various radiologic services and central laboratories of microbiology and biochemistry.

Hospital medicine differs from public health practice in that its focus is on the sick individual who is in need of special medical care. Related to the inpatient units, the hospital also includes consultant services, outpatient care, and emergency services, all of which are concerned with special categories of patients. However, hospital medicine does extend to the care of well individuals, as in obstetrics and neonatal pediatrics. While these specialties focus much of their skill on well individuals in general, the clinical medicine practiced in hospitals is essentially disease-oriented. The scope and methods of history taking, physical examination, and investigations involving special laboratory, roentgenologic, and other examinations have been systematized for each of the different specialties.

Hospital Catchment Areas and Primary Care

The catchment area of a major general hospital often varies according to the specialty and the frequency of occurrence of cases cared for by the specialty. The term "catchment population" perhaps reflects the reality more accurately than catchment area, especially when we realize that the catchment populations for different specialties of a hospital vary according to such factors as age and sex and the specific conditions for which the department caters. It may be expected that the catchment population for inpatient care will generally be much larger for specialties such as neurology and neurosurgery than for internal medicine and general surgery. It is also important to remember that some services of a hospital, such as outpatient clinics and emergency rooms, are used as primary-care facilities by many people. This is especially so in the center of large cities, where many of the major teaching hospitals of developed countries are located. It is even a more striking feature of large hospitals located in the growing cities of many developing countries, which cater to the primary medical care demands of masses of people from the city itself and from rural communities. This extensive use of emergency facilities and outpatient departments of city hospitals has become a major problem for the organization of medical care. They epitomize the depersonalization of primary health care. Hence, their impact may actually be detrimental. Of much relevance to our considerations of health care in the community are hospitals that have links with various types of community health centers or clinics. In some areas, decentralized clinics and dispensaries are the direct responsibility of a hospital. Such decentralized hospital clinics are a means of extending the catchment area of the hospital to include communities that do not have any other modern medical services.

Another development from the hospital has been the home care of patients who can be adequately treated at home if there is ready access to hospital when needed.[2]

The impact that these major institutions of modern medical care have on a community's health is not readily measured. It is probably considerably less than that of environmental and public health services. Serious questions are being raised increasingly as to the contribution of modern medicine to the decline in mortality and morbidity and the improvement of the population's health. Is the present-day vast investment of finance, resources, and technology justified? This will be discussed later in this chapter.

PUBLIC HEALTH PRACTICE

The public health movement is one of the major elements of social action, aimed at modifying the environment and people's behavior in order to promote the health and welfare of society. Its origins lie deep in the traditions of all societies, but its scientific development is comparatively recent. It is linked with the technologic and industrial revolution, and with advances in knowledge of the environment and of people. The main objectives of public health practice are to promote health, prevent disease, and ensure the best possible distribution of health and medical care facilities. In placing greater emphasis on its promotive and preventive objectives than on curative care, it stresses the importance of modifying the environment, health-related behavior, and health action by the community.

Outstanding in the contribution that public health makes to the community's health are various environmental health services, nutrition programs, communicable disease control, and personal preventive services, especially maternal and child health care. Organized on a national scale, with a citywide or regional basis, the environmental services involve major projects for the sanitary control of air, water, and food supplies and thereby prevent the occurrence of many communicable and other diseases. Similarly, protective measures against environmental hazards, such as noise, light, and pollution, are central features of industrial health.

Nutrition programs have also been focused on the needs of important segments of the population in a country as a whole or in a particular region. Thus, national health education may be directed toward increasing or decreasing the consumption of particular foods according to availability and changing knowledge of nutrition. Action may also be taken by means of subsidies, taxation, or special food fortification measures. Among the earliest successful examples of the modification of foods was the use of iodized salt in the prevention of endemic goiter. This was followed by the equally imaginative fluoridation of water supplies for the reduction of dental caries, by bread enrichment, and by recent experiments in Latin America using sugar fortified with vitamin A for the prevention of blindness and other complications of vitamin A deficiency.[3] Other important measures have included special provision for promoting the nutritional status of selected groups, such as school milk and school meal services in many countries and "meals-on-wheels" programs for the elderly at home.

Mass Health Examinations

These have a relatively long history and a well-established place in public health practice. Widespread public health programs often include mass screening methods for finding cases of communicable diseases affecting large numbers of people. Such diseases include malaria, syphilis, yaws, leprosy, tuberculosis, smallpox, and trachoma. Initiated as part of the public health movement, these measures have been extended to vast areas of the world. Where relevant, the survey includes investigation of vectors and various conditions that facilitate transmission and occurrence of the disease. The purpose of these surveys include case finding, surveillance of infection, and intervention for its control. A dramatic result of such an approach was the total eradication of smallpox, as announced by the World Health Organization (WHO) in 1977.

Surveys of growth and nutritional state also have a long history. One hundred years ago, Bowditch demonstrated an association between the height and weight of Boston schoolchildren and socioeconomic status.[4,5] This association between physical growth in children and their nutritional status is so consistent that measurements of growth are recommended as objective indices of the nutritional status of population groups. Surveys of diet and nutrition are now widespread and updated; standardized methods for such examinations have been published periodically by WHO.[6,7] The purposes of these surveys are similar to those concerned with communicable diseases, in this case the promotion of health and more satisfactory growth by means of improved diet and nutrition.

Maternal and Child Health Care

Public health action of the kind we have discussed has most often been conducted away from personal health care, especially community-based primary health care. The major exceptions to this are maternal and child health services, which are often conducted in special neighborhood or village health centers. Where they exist they are among the most important primary health care services in the community. As an instrument of the public health movement, the origin of the clinic goes back to the establishment of infant welfare centers in France and England in the nineteenth century. During the twentieth century, neighborhood maternal and child health centers became a widespread feature of the public health services in cities and rural areas. Staffed by specially trained public health nurses (health visitors), medically qualified child health officers, and sometimes visited by pediatricians and obstetricians, such centers conduct a promotive and preventive service for mothers and children. They carry out pre- and postnatal examinations of mothers, health and developmental examinations of children, immunizations, health education of parents, and referral for special care where necessary. In addition, mother and child centers are often the base from which public health nurses undertake home visits for maternal and infant health supervision and for visiting the families of school-children under their care. More recently, these centers have been expanding their public health functions to include such activities as family spacing, health supervision of the elderly, and care of the chronically sick and disabled. Where these services are well developed, the mother and child center has, in fact, expanded to a preventive and promotive family health care center.

Public Health and Clinical Medicine

The focus of public health is on the population group rather than the individual. It is in this perhaps more than in any other feature that it differs from clinical medicine, a difference that is reflected in its history taking, methods of examination of a problem, diagnosis, action, and evaluation. Its history taking is in reality an epidemiologic study of health trends in relation to changes in the community and its environment. Its examination involves both the direct health examination of groups of individuals and the gathering of data from various sources, such as death records and the records of hospitals, clinics, and school health services. Analysis of these data provides the basis for diagnosis of the state of health of the population. This includes mortality and morbidity rates and their differential distribution, as well as more direct indicators of health, such as outcome of pregnancy, differences in growth and development of various groups of children, and the functioning and daily activities of older people in the population. Public health action is directed toward improvement of the environment, national food consumption, living and working conditions, ways of rearing children, and other health-promotive activities. In evaluation of its actions, we are concerned with ensuring that what should be done is being done and that this is having the desired effects on the health of the population as a whole or on those groups to which the program has been directed.

The public health and hospital services just described are examples of primary care, which are extensions of these major institutions to what they regard as the periphery. The decision-making authorities are themselves seldom in direct contact with the communities to which their services are extended. The larger the institution, the more likely is its administration to be separated from the people, especially the small communities whose members use its outreach facilities. This inevitably leads to separation from the community of what should be essentially a personal and community service, thus allowing little scope for informal and ongoing community participation and little or no role for communities in the development of their own health care.

There is, too, increasing involvement of national governments in personal health care. This extension of responsibility for the public's health from regional or local authorities to the central government is well organized.[8,9] In this process, the responsible authorities are still further removed from the individual, family, and small community, with the consequent lack of involvement in decision making by those most directly affected by the services.

PRIMARY HEALTH CARE IN THE COMMUNITY

As usually understood, primary health care involves the practitioner to whom a person first turns when ill or when seeking advice on personal health. Such a practice may include patients of all ages, both sexes, with any illness, disability, or other perceived health need. In the Western world, the main community-based primary-care practitioners are physicians and nurses. The practice of primary-care physicians may include promotive, preventive, curative, and alleviative functions, but their dominant function is care of the ill or disabled patient. Although oriented toward the needs of the individual, their practice often involves the family and others who are closely associated with the patient. This extension to the family has been a feature of European and American medicine, and the terms general practitioner (GP) and family physician are often used synonymously. It is not always realized in Western society that the general practitioner or family physician is not the traditional doctor in other societies. Furthermore, primary health care is undergoing change, in response to technologic advances and specialization in medicine. It is extending to include other professional and auxiliary health personnel. The solo physician-practitioner is being succeeded by group practice and the health team. The community nurse is much involved in primary health care, and many approaches to the doctor-nurse team in community practice have been reported. Specialization has raised the potential for some aspects of health care and at the same time created problems in the provision of primary care. Specialists in pediatrics, psychiatry, and internal medicine often provide primary medical care and may work in group practice or in community health centers. Even more narrowly defined specialties may be involved in primary medical care, including obstetrics, ophthalmology, ENT (ear, nose, and throat), and sometimes those concerned with care of patients with long-term illness. Neurologists, cardiologists, and other specialists may be in fact, if not in name, the personal primary physicians of patients who are under their care for a long-term illness. While they have this role, their special experience has not prepared them for it. Unfortunately, this is true too of the primary-care physician whose practice is based on the clinical training obtained in teaching hospitals.

It is by means of experience in primary care itself and training for it that practitioners must develop the special skills needed for this type of practice. These require special emphasis on the social, cultural, and behavioral aspects of the patient's history and life situation, including their various health-relevant habits and perceptions of illness. Another important feature of primary care in the community is its continuity over long periods of time; this builds a special relationship between practitioners, patients, and their families. Focus on the family is central for primary care, since it is a determinant of the health of its individual members and the most important institution in health care. Primary-care practitioners who come to know several members of the same family in the course of their daily practice are more able to use their knowledge of family resources, relationships, and perception of health in the care of individuals in the family. However, it is the exception rather than the rule for physicians to be sophisticated in this aspect of their practice.

In addition to the medical and public health services provided in the community by primary-care physicians and nurses, health care in the community often includes: midwifery at clinics and at home, dentistry, pharmacy, optometry, chiropody, adult and child psychiatry, physiotherapy, and occupational therapy. Various social services working with the same people may have a close relationship with health services in the neighborhood community.

In response to the relative neglect of primary care in the community compared with hospital medicine, there has been a resurgence of interest in the education of primary-care physicians and other practitioners. The neglect was, and still is, part of the process of specialization in hospital medicine. With medical practice becoming more specialized and increasingly hospital centered, until very recently there has been little investment in education for primary care in undergraduate and postgraduate medical education. In some areas, there is already a maldistribution of physicians—an excess of surgeons and other specialists and a lack of primary-care physicians.[10-12]

The shortage of primary-care physicians can be met in several ways. Family physicians, general internists, and pediatricians may be trained for primary care, but this will mean a reduction in the number of internists who are being trained for subspecialties.[13,14] Even if this problem is solved (and it is doubtful that it will be), there remain other perhaps more important questions. Is the effort really worthwhile? Is the problem only one of the distribution of doctors? Perhaps it is more fundamental and involves the need for reorientation of medicine as a whole.

Medical services have become an outstanding feature of modern society, especially in the developed countries. The growth of these services requires considerable investment of finance, manpower, and technology. The work of serious students of health, economics, and society challenges the wisdom of this process.[15-21]Changes in the environment, standards of education, and social status as determined by occupation, education, and income exert greater influence than does the medical care system on favorable mortality and morbidity trends, as well as on improvements in health. In a recent study comparing the mortality rates in 18 developed countries, little relationship was found with medical care facilities, such as the prevalence of doctors, nurses, and acute hospital beds.[19] Furthermore, it is not the highly complicated and expensive technology that makes the greatest contribution. Thus, the widespread use of relatively cheap advances, namely the antibiotics, has had a considerable effect on reducing mortality since World War II.[16]

COMMUNITY-ORIENTED
PRIMARY HEALTH CARE

The skills of the primary-care practitioner should be based on a holistic concept of individual, family, and community health. This requires a reorientation in our thinking about health and health care.

We have given separate consideration to several services that contribute to health care of the community, namely, hospital services, public health practice, and primary health care in the community. These services are often separately provided by different agencies, none of which focuses on health care of the small community as distinct from care of the individual patient in hospital or primary medical care, and public health control measures at a regional or national level. Thus, while there is universal provision of some form of primary medical care in the community, little attention has been given to the development of its potential for promoting the community's health as a whole. Practical experience in community health care has had little place in the teaching of medical students or even in the activities of schools of public health. However, some aspects of community health care are now beginning to receive more attention in a number of countries, a movement that is being actively sponsored by the World Health Organization. The first international conference on primary health care took place in Alma Ata, U.S.S.R., in 1978.[22,23]

The move toward a union of the previously separated preventive and curative services was reflected in various proposals and activities after World War I, in the United States, the United Kingdom, and the newly formed U.S.S.R. Among the cornerstones of these proposals was the concept of the comprehensive health center. Terris, an exponent of the advantages of the comprehensive health center, states that in 1919, Dr. H. Biggs, commissioner of health of New York State, made the first proposal for state aid to local health centers, which would include the traditional local authority public health services, curative medical and surgical clinics, and hospital facilities. While these proposals were not accepted, they represent the extent to which leaders in public health at that time were already pressing for a redefinition of public health that would widen its scope.[24,25]

At the same time, in 1920, the Dawson Report on Medical and

Allied Services in England and Wales was published.[26] Some of the recommendations of that report are highly relevant to the present time. It recommended that preventive and curative medicine not be separated in any scheme of medical services and that they should be included in the work of general practitioners, whose duties should involve them in "communal as well as individual medicine" carried out within health centers.

In the U.S.S.R., the health center combining curative and preventive services was an early feature of health care in factories and in residential neighborhoods.[27] In other less developed countries, too, there were important explorations of this kind. Among the most innovative experiments of that time was that of John Grant, who in 1921 was appointed as head of the department of hygiene of the Peking Union Medical College in China, which had been taken over by the Rockefeller Foundation. Based on his argument that preventive medicine must be provided with facilities comparable with those of the hospital, he established a "demonstration health station" in Peking. In this center, health maintenance and preventive and curative medicine were brought together and used in the teaching of medical and nursing undergraduate students and public health nurses. This must surely have been a pioneer development of the field training area. Grant's subsequent career and influence in many countries have been studied by Seipp.[28-30]

During the past 40 years, various forms of the community health center have become widespread as institutions for providing a variety of health services within communities, in urban neighborhoods, and in rural villages. This holds true for the more developed as well as the developing countries of the world. However even those places that have coordinated curative and preventive services tend to confine themselves to clinical practice rather than a system of health care that unifies individual and community medicine, namely community-oriented primary health care.

Community health care involves activities toward the promotion of health of the community, together with efforts to prevent disease, to treat and care for the sick, and contribute toward the rehabilitation of disabled people in the community. The focus is on the health of the community as a whole by intervention at the individual and group level. The concept of a unified practice of community medicine and primary health care thus includes both clinical and public health activities.

Primary care of the individual has already been discussed, especially those forms of primary care that are based in the community. Further consideration of community medicine is desirable before dealing with its role in developing community-oriented primary health care.

Community Medicine

Community medicine has grown out of public health and medical administration. It is a useful new term, which recognizes the recent developments taking place in public health, health care planning, and administration. Like public health, it deals with population groups rather than the individual patient. In the present context, it is distinguished from other forms of personal health care in the community in that its interest is centered on the community as a whole and the groups of which communities are composed. Community medicine requires scientific foundations for action. Diagnosis of the state of health of a community is as important for community medicine as clinical diagnosis is for the care of an individual patient. It also needs to ensure continuing surveillance of the population's health and evaluation of health care programs. This requires knowledge of epidemiology and skills for its application in practice, biostatistics, and an understanding of the social sciences, especially in their application to epidemiology, health-relevant behavior of communities, community health care, and health administration. In Great Britain, community medicine has recently been recognized as a specialty. The Faculty of Community Medicine was established by the Royal College of Physicians in 1972. It has defined community medicine as a branch of medicine concerned with populations or groups rather than with individual patients, requiring special knowledge of epidemiology, organization and evaluation of medical care, and the medical aspects of health service administration. The faculty's definition extends to include well-established fields of social and preventive medicine, such as health education and rehabilitation.[31]

Practitioners of community medicine need to answer the following cardinal questions:

1. What is the state of health of the community?
2. What are the factors responsible for this state of health?
3. What is being done about it by the health service system and by the community itself?
4. What more can be done, what is proposed, and what is the expected outcome?
5. What measures are needed to continue health surveillance of the community and to evaluate the effects of what is being done?

Answers to these questions are related to each of the important areas of community medicine; namely, community diagnosis, community health care, surveillance of health, and evaluation of the programs developed.

Community Diagnosis.   Answers to the first two closely related questions—What is the state of health of the community and what are the determinants of this state of health?—are basically the function of epidemiology, which is defined as the study of the distribution of any health condition in a population and the determinants of this distribution.

Community Health Care.   In planning the action to be taken (Question 4), we need to consider not only the community diagnosis but also what is already being done by the community itself and by existing health services (Question 3).

Surveillance and Evaluation.   The last of the basic questions facing practitioners of community medicine (Question 5) are functions of epidemiology and biostatistics. For this purpose, a system of health recording and data analysis is needed to ensure ready retrieval of information on the activities being undertaken and the state of health of the community.

Now that we have reviewed the scope of community medicine, further consideration will be given to the unified practice of community medicine and primary health care. What should be the essential characteristics of such community health care?

It should be community-based, community-oriented, and the community should be involved. The health care should be coordinated with other activities in the community that have relevance for health and welfare (horizontal coordination). It also needs to be coordinated with the broader system of health services of the region and country (vertical coordination), and its various activities should be well supported by the major public health and hospital services. It needs considerable investment of resources, and as emphasized by the director general of WHO, it should have top priority in this respect: "Problems of the periphery should determine the content and organization of the more central levels of the health system whereas it is usually just the opposite."[32]

Community-Based Health Care

The main concern of community health care is with communities such as those found in blocks of buildings and neighborhoods of cities, in small towns and rural villages, and in groups within these communities, which include families, schools, places of work, and residential institutions. Thus, it is concerned with the health care of relatively small communities, their families, and other primary groups.

Why this emphasis on the location of the service in the community? We have seen that major hospitals and public health agencies provide primary-care services, which are heavily used by the public. Useful as such services may be, they are lacking in several respects, the most important of which is perhaps the relationship between the staff and the population using the service. When services are located within the community, the number of people for whom a particular health team is responsible can be relatively well defined. The size of the population will vary according to the density of living in the locality. The higher the density, the greater the number of people that can be incorporated within the scope of the health center practice. However, for better care one health team should be required to cater to only a section of that population. Thus, in an urban neighborhood with a high-density population, a health center might be composed of a number of health teams; in a rural area, a single health team might have to cover a wider area, with its team members traveling out to different points from a center, or being stationed at several subcenters in the area.

So far we have emphasized two desirable attributes of a community health care service, nearness and smallness. The service should be so located that mothers with babies in baby carriages or strollers and older or disabled people are within easy walking distance. Thus all persons should have ready access to the center for health care, as well as for attending group discussions or community meetings. The homes should also be near enough to ensure easy access by members of the health team for home care of the sick, family discussions, health education, and regular visiting in the various preventive and promotive programs.

The importance of each health care team working with a small population is that it facilitates an ongoing, friendly, and relatively informal contact between members of the health team and the community.[33] At the same time, such a community served by the health team may itself be essentially a primary group in the sense in which Cooley first described primary groups many years ago.[34] They are characterized by frequent or ongoing face-to-face contacts and include such groups as the family, the neighborhood, children's play groups, and other informal friendship groups.

The advantage of such primary relationships is the encouragement of community participation in the development of its health care. The individuals' acquaintance with one another can lead to a type of representation in which the elected representatives are known to almost everyone within the community. In this way, more distant and formal representation is avoided in such a personal community service, and barriers between the health team and community prevented.

The advantages of a community based health service are:

1. Ability to promote primary relationships between the community and the health team, thereby enabling health care to proceed in the framework of an easy, ongoing relationship between different members of the team and the community, promoting community involvement in acceptance of responsibility for the health program, and facilitating the health team's awareness of meaningful events and happenings in the community and its families.
2. By ensuring nearness of the center to the homes in the community, it facilitates visits to the health center by members of the community and ease of access by members of the health team to homes.
3. By defining the area of responsibility of the health center, it is simpler to define the community in terms of its demography and other attributes and to identify the families and individuals who are eligible for care by different members of the health team.

Community-Oriented Care

In planning community health care, we need answers to questions such as whether there are sufficient meeting points between the existing separate health services. If the services were integrated, would this help in promoting the community's health and at the same time improve the care of individual patients? With these ends in mind, the features of health care that can be united would appear to be those that are community-oriented and based in the local community. Thus, the following types of practitioners might be brought together:

Clinicians providing curative care in the community, whether they are general family physicians, pediatricians, internists, nurse practitioners, or nurses caring for sick patients at home.

Practitioners involved in public health practice, such as maternal and infant health care and schoolchild health services. These include community physicians and community health nurses, such as public health nurses and health visitors.

Sanitarians, especially those in rural areas, who control the village water supply, refuse disposal, and agricultural hygiene, involving them in much contact with people in their homes and at work.

In this way, community health care can combine the different elements of health care of individuals, their families, and the community. This requires an extension of responsibility of practitioners to health care of the community as well as of the individuals who seek care.

The scope of local community health care in a combined practice of this kind will now be considered.

Health Care of Individuals and Families in the Community

This involves primary and secondary care facilities.

Primary Care.   This includes curative and preventive personal services.

Curative services:
Comprehensive care of illness readily treated at neighborhood clinics or at home.
Initial care and referral for more complicated conditions requiring further investigation or treatment.
Home care of the chronic sick with physical or mental illness.
Aftercare of patients discharged from hospital.

Preventive and promotive personal health services:
Family spacing.
Pre- and postnatal care of mothers.
Infant and young child care.
School health services.
Immunizations.

In addition, primary preventive personal services are now extending to include mental health services, preventive cardiology, and health care for the aged and disabled.

While there are still many places in which curative and preventive services are provided separately in the same neighborhoods or villages, there is growing acceptance of the desirability of bringing them together. Different approaches have been used to achieve this objective. The importance of continuing personal care by a personal doctor, a family nurse, or other practitioner is agreed on by almost all students of health and medical care. The desirability of a single health team being responsible for both preventive and curative care is thus more readily appreciated. Patient-doctor relationships and their continuity have received much attention.[35-37] There is need for further study of such relationships of the health team with individuals, their families, and the community.[38]

Secondary Health Care.   The main responsibility for secondary care is that of hospitals and other consultative or specialist clinics. The common procedure is referral of a patient by a primary-care practitioner for further investigation or treatment. However, there are situations in which the secondary-care specialist, such as an obstetrician-gynecologist, psychiatrist, cardiologist, or orthopedist, might improve the service by joining with the primary-care team. Home care of disabled patients and their families is often rendered more effective by the availability of physiotherapists and occupational therapists on the staff of a hospital or secondary-care clinic. Similarly, other facilities of a hospital can add considerably to the scope of work of primary-care centers, for example, by providing special laboratory procedures for which the health center sends the required specimens so that the patients themselves do not have to go to the hospital.

Community Medicine in Primary Health Care.   The scope of community medicine when linked with primary health care for a relatively small community needs further consideration. The activities would be focused on physical and mental health status of the community, as well as its social well-being, but in order to develop community medicine in the framework of primary health care decisions about priorities have to be made. These decisions will depend on the kind of community the health center serves, its state of health, the skills and interests of the health team, and the priority rating the community gives to various aspects of its health. Depending on these factors, the community programs may include one or more of the following areas:

Promotion of Health:
Reproduction: by appropriate programs for family planning and maternity care.
Growth and development: by programs for infant and child care, including nutrition, health education, and promotion of social interaction.
Aging: by programs on physical activity, diet, and social functioning.

Prevention of disease and disability:
Communicable disease: immunization, sanitation of the immediate environment, protection of food and water.

Malnutrition: health education and feeding schemes for the prevention of the common malnutrition syndromes in the community.

Accidents and injuries: home, school, and neighborhood, surveillance of hazards.

Noncommunicable diseases: personal behavior, such as diet, smoking, and physical activity directed toward prevention of various disorders.

Care of the Sick and Disabled.   In addition to general clinics for ambulatory patients, special programs may be arranged for home care of housebound patients and for particular groups of disorders such as heart disease, stroke, hypertension, and diabetes.

If community medicine and primary health care are to be brought together in the health care of local communities, we must ensure that doctors, nurses, and other members of the team are trained for this purpose. The team should have knowledge of epidemiology and community diagnosis no less than it has in examination and diagnosis of individuals. In addition to its skills in the treatment of patients, it needs the skills for action that will affect the health of the community as a whole, or its subgroups. These skills should include health education, community organization, and promotion of family and community involvement in health activities. While not all members of the team can be expected to have the same qualifications, in level or in kind, the team as a whole must possess the various skills needed to develop the unified practice of primary health care and community medicine.

The usual training of medical and nursing students does not prepare them for the tasks envisaged, and thus new orientations and fresh approaches are needed. The development of new forms of community health care involves consideration of the complementary functions of clinical and epidemiologic skills in their application to the care of individuals and to group or community oriented health action. Table 1-1 lists the corresponding components of clinical and epidemiologic skills in community-oriented primary health care.

Community Involvement

In care of the individual, the patient's compliance with advice is often central to the success of the treatment, especially in cases needing medication over long periods of time. For example, one of the first measures of effectiveness of a program to control hypertension on a community-wide basis is the extent of compliance with the recommendations. Are the hypertensive patients taking the medications pre-

TABLE 1-1

Summary of the Complementary Functions of Clinical and Epidemiologic Skills in Development of Community-Oriented Primary Health Care

CLINICAL (Individual)	EPIDEMIOLOGIC (Population Group)
Examination of a patient Interview and examination of individuals by history taking, physical and psychologic examinations, laboratory, x-ray, and other special techniques.	Survey State of health of community and families, using questionnaires, physical and psychologic testing, and special facilities for such investigations.
Diagnosis 1. Usually of a patient. Differential diagnosis to determine main causes of patient's complaint.	Community Diagnosis 1. Usually problem-oriented. Differential distribution of a particular condition in the community and the causes of this distribution.
2. Appraisal of health status of a "well" person, such as a pregnant woman, well children, periodic health examinations of adults.	2. Health status of the community as a whole or of defined segments of it, e.g., health of expectant mothers, growth and development of children, birth and death rates.
Treatment 1. According to diagnosis and depending on resources of patient and medical institutions.	Treatment 1. According to the community diagnosis and depending on resources of the health service system.
2. Intervention usually follows on the patient seeking care for illness or advice about health.	2. Intervention on basis of survey findings often before any illness notified or recognized.
Continuing observation Evaluation of patient's progress and sometimes for further diagnostic work-up.	Continuing surveillance Surveillance of health state of community and ensuring continuing action. Evaluation of intervention programs.

scribed? Was the patient seeking care because of illness, or was the initiative that of the health service through a screening survey locating individuals with high blood pressure readings? Was the screening survey conducted by the personal doctor as part of his/her practice, or was it a mass screening survey organized by an impersonal health authority? The answers to these questions would surely influence the patient's response to advice and hence compliance with a medication regime.

The individual's sovereignty is involved in these decisions for action in his or her own interest. Recognition of this simple but fundamental truth would lead practitioners to give more attention to patients' perception of their health condition and the possible effects of treatment.

While participation in decision making by the individual patient is important for satisfactory care, it is perhaps even more so in community health care. There have been a number of reports on the failure of health and other development programs that were not acceptable to the communities concerned.[39-44] The failures have been more readily observed in cross-cultural situations, where the health team aimed to produce change in communities whose way of life, technology, and value system differed markedly from their own. Their enthusiasm in attaining their objectives was often not matched by their understanding of the community and hence their sensitivity to the possible adverse reactions that might be generated by their activities.

There is, therefore, an increasing acceptance of the need for community involvement in the initiation and provision of community health care. What does this mean for the health team and for the community's health? Understanding the community is essential for a health team that will be expected to work with, and encourage the active participation of, the community in its own health care. If the basic education of team members has not included community health, they should be given the opportunity for special study with those epidemiologists, health educators, and behavioral scientists who have a special interest in the application of their disciplines to the structure and health of communities and their health care.

The way in which communities function has been studied by many social scientists, but such investigations have not yet been accepted as an integral part of community health care. A health care team should have knowledge of social health relevance, such as community networks of relationships, occupations and activities of daily living, family structure and kinship in the community, and its formal and informal leadership. Each situation in which a member of the health team meets with an individual or group offers an opportunity for such observations. Furthermore, community health surveys of knowledge, attitudes, and practices (KAP) can be planned in association with members of the community and sometimes conducted by them.

Perhaps the most important prerequisite for satisfactory functioning of a community in its own health care is a relationship of basic trust between the community and the health team. The respect the health team gives to the community will determine the team's attitude to the prevailing beliefs and health care practices. The community health council of a neighborhood or village health center will develop into an effective advisory and involved group only if its representativeness is well accepted by the community and the professional health team.

Recognition of the gulf that sometimes separates professional health workers from the people to whom they deliver care has resulted in the appointment of members of the community to bridge the gap.[45-47] Community health workers of this kind may be selected by the community from among its own members.[48] They may remain responsible to the community without becoming members of the staff of a health center, and function as a bridge from the community to the health team, representing the community and interpreting the needs of the patients, families, or groups. On the other hand, they might become members of the health team and be given special training to enable them to expand their functions to health education and community organization. Such specially trained health workers who are members of the community can themselves stimulate community involvement in various projects and in the conduct of the health program as a whole.

If health is about the quality of life, promoting community involvement is not only for the purpose of achieving specific goals such as building protected water supplies or changing food production and diet. Community involvement is in itself a health activity, promotive of social well-being and mental health. The sense of being able to influence one's own community's development is perhaps the essential difference between "development" and "being developed." This is perhaps more applicable to communities alienated from the dominant social, cultural, and economic classes, among whom anomie is widespread. Perhaps the more the community is removed from the mainstream of modern technology and medical care, the more important it is to encourage community participation and acceptance of responsibility for its health care.

Community involvement in health activities varies in different communities, related not only to the decision making of the health team, but also to the nature of the community. It requires the organization of groups in the community with special interests in various health problems or in health maintenance. This needs the systematic approach of community organization.[49-51] It is an activity that has been given much emphasis in recent developments of community health care. The neighborhood health centers that followed the civil rights movement of the 1960s in the United States emphasized the central role of the community itself in their development.[52-58] Community health action has become a feature of the primary care approach now being advocated by the World Health Organization and the United Nations Children's Fund (UNICEF),[22,23] and an increasing number of countries in Asia, Europe, the Americas, and Africa.[45,59-63] It is often said that community health care of the kind being discussed cannot be developed in metropolitan city communities, especially in the city centers. Has not the way of life in such centers altered so profoundly as to render traditional sense of community nonexistent? The success of the musical *Fiddler on the Roof* is perhaps worth recalling. Based on the original Yiddish novel, *Tevye, The Milkman*, by Sholom Aleichem, this musical carried the story of the traditional Jewish family and community of the Eastern European *shtetl* (village) to the major metropolitan centers of the world. Its widespread acclaim among apparently differing peoples in these centers suggests that metropolitan men and women of different sociocultural origins share much with one another and with their forebears. Beneath their liberation from the village with its mores resides perhaps a sense of community and a yen for the network of primary relationships with its meaningful bonds.

It is in big cities, and especially in the inner-city areas, that community-based, community-oriented services are needed to replace the emergency room and outpatient services of large hospitals as general primary care facilities. It is true that there are a number of activities that do not take place in the locality of living. People commute considerable distances to their work as well as for shopping, to school, and other purposes. However, it is important to list some of the local activities that may be seen in the neighborhoods or streets of big cities: mothers wheeling their infants in baby carriages, people chatting in the streets and shops, children's play groups, children going to nursery schools and elementary schools, and the aged and disabled walking to and from various places. Neighborhood health centers are of special use to these groups and need to adapt their programs to the characteristics of the community. They would also serve important sections of the population living in the area if they were open at times that are convenient for workers and students returning home in the late afternoons and evenings.

Planning often proceeds from the center out to the periphery. Whatever advantages this may have for the planning of cities and their suburban areas, and this is questioned, it loses in respect of community health care. The centrally situated hospitals or public health institutes are unsuited to the task of providing basic primary and community health care to the many communities in the region they serve. Relatively small neighborhood or village communities have little opportunity to participate in the decision making of these larger institutions, which should rather be seen as backup facilities for community health centers, in which the community may more readily be involved and the individual less easily dwarfed.

REFERENCES

1. Levitt R: The Reorganised National Health Service, 2nd ed. London, Croom Helm, 1977.
2. Cherkasky M: The Montefiore hospital home care program. Am J Public Health 39:29, 1949.
3. World Health Organization: Nutrition News. WHO Chron 32:475, 1978.
4. Bowditch HP: The Growth of Children. Annual Reports of the Massachusetts State Board of Health, 1877, 1879.
5. Roberts LJ: Nutrition Work with Children. Chicago, Univ. of Chicago Press, 1935, chap 4.
6. Jelliffe DB: The Assessment of the Nutritional Status of the Community. Geneva, World Health Organization, Monograph Series No. 53, 1966.
7. Waterlow JC, Buzina R, Keller W, et al.: The presentation and use of height and weight data for comparing the nutritional status of groups of children under the age of 10 years. Bull WHO 55:489, 1977.
8. Rosen G: A History of Public Health. New York, MD Publications, 1958.
9. Sheps CG (chairman): Higher Education for Public Health. Report of Milbank Memorial Fund Commission. New York, Milbank Memorial Fund, 1976.
10. Institute of Medicine: A Manpower Policy for Primary Health Care. Washington, D.C., National Academy of Sciences, 1978.
11. Scheffler RM, Weisfeld N, Ruby G, et al.: A manpower policy for primary health care. N Engl J Med 298:1058, 1978.
12. Relman AS: Who will train all those primary-care physicians? N Engl J Med 299:652, 1978.
13. Perkoff GT: General internal medicine, family practice or something better? N Engl J Med 299:654, 1978.
14. Colwill JM: Primary-care education in multiple specialties. N Engl J Med 299:657, 1978.
15. Fuchs VR: Who Shall Live? New York, Basic, 1974.
16. ———: Economics, health, and post-industrial society. Milbank Mem Fund Q 57:153, 1979.
17. Illich I: Medical Nemesis. New York, Pantheon, 1976.
18. McKeown T: The Role of Medicine: Dream, Mirage or Nemesis? London, Nuffield Provincial Hospitals Trust, 1976.
19. Cochrane AL, St. Leger AS, Moore F: Health service "input" and mortality "output" in developed countries. J Epidemiol Community Health 32:200, 1978.
20. Knowles JH (ed): Doing Better and Feeling Worse: Health in the United States. New York, Norton, 1977.
21. Bradshaw JS: Doctors on Trial. London, Wildwood House, 1979.
22. Joint Report of World Health Organization and United Nations

Children's Fund: Primary Health Care. Geneva and New York, WHO and UNICEF, 1978.

23. Report of the International Conference on Primary Health Care, Alma-Ata, U.S.S.R., 1978. Geneva, WHO, 1978.

24. Terris M: Hermann Biggs' contribution to the modern concept of the health center. Bull Hist Med 20:387, 1946.

25. ——: The comprehensive health center. Public Health Rep 78:861, 1963.

26. Dawson Report: Consultative Council on Medical and Allied Services (chairman, Lord Dawson of Penn) Interim Report on the Future Provision of Medical and Allied Services. London, HMSO, 1920.

27. Sigerist HE: Socialised Medicine in the Soviet Union. London, Gollancz, 1937.

28. Seipp C: Health Care for the Community. Baltimore, Johns Hopkins Press, 1963.

29. ——: John B. Grant 1890–1962 (personal communication).

30. ——: Excerpts from John Grant's First Annual Report of the Peking Demonstration Health Station 1925–1926 (personal communication).

31. Parry WH: Community medicine. Community Health 4:23, 1972.

32. Mahler H: Blueprint for Health for All. WHO Chron 31:491, 1977.

33. Schumacher EF: Small Is Beautiful. London, Blond & Briggs, 1973.

34. Cooley HC: Social Organization. New York, Schocken, 1962 (first published in 1909, Scribner's).

35. Balint M: The Doctor, His Patient and the Illness. New York, Universities Press, 1957.

36. Hulka BS, Kupper LJ, Cassel JC, et al.: Practice characteristics and quality of primary medical care: the doctor-patient relationship. Med Care 13:808, 1975.

37. Ornstein PH: The family physician as a "therapeutic instrument." J Fam Pract 4:659, 1977.

38. Marsh G, Kaim-Candle P: Team Care in General Practice. London, Croom Helm, 1976.

39. Spicer EH (ed): Human Problems in Technological Change. New York, Russell Sage Foundation, 1952.

40. Saunders L: Cultural Differences and Medical Care: The Care of the Spanish-Speaking People of the Southwest. New York, Russell Sage Foundation, 1954.

41. Paul BD (ed): Health, Culture and Community. New York, Russell Sage Foundation, 1955.

42. Foster GM: Traditional Cultures: and the Impact of Technological Change. New York, Harper & Row, 1962.

43. Foster GM: Applied Anthropology. Boston, Little, Brown, 1969.

44. Glasser R: The Net and the Quest. Patterns of Community and How They Can Survive Progress. London, Temple Smith, 1977.

45. Kark SL, Steuart GW: A Practice of Social Medicine. Edinburgh, Livingstone, 1962.

46. Zahn S: Neighborhood medical care demonstration training program. Milbank Mem Fund Q 46:309, 1968.

47. Adair J, Deuschle KW: The People's Health: Anthropology and Medicine in a Navajo Community. New York, Appleton, 1970.

48. McNeur RW: The Changing Roles and Education of Health Care Person-

nel Worldwide in View of the Increase of Basic Health Services. Philadelphia, Society for Health and Human Values, 1978.

49. Ross MG: Community Organization: Theory and Principles. New York, Harper, 1955.
50. Wise HB, Levin LS, Kurahara RT: Community development and health education: I. Community organization as a health tactic. Milbank Mem Fund Q 46:329, 1968.
51. Coe RM, Pepper M: Community Medicine. Some New Perspectives. New York, McGraw-Hill, 1978.
52. Gibson CD: The Neighborhood health center: the primary unit of health care. Am J Public Health 58:1188, 1968.
53. Geiger JH: The neighborhood health center: education of the faculty in preventive medicine. Arch Environ Health 14:912, 1967.
54. Geiger JH: A health center in Mississippi—a case study in social medicine. In Corey L, Saltman SE, Epstein MF (eds): Medicine in a Changing Society. St. Louis, Mosby, 1971, pp 157–167.
55. Hatch J: Community shares in policy decisions for a rural health center. Hospitals 43:109, 1969.
56. Stokes A, Banta D, Putnam S: The Columbia Point Health Association evolution of a community health board. Am J Public Health 62:1229, 1972.
57. Bellin SS, Geiger HJ: Actual public acceptance of the neighborhood health center by the urban poor. JAMA 214:2147, 1970.
58. Wise HB: Montefiore Hospital neighborhood medical care demonstration. Milbank Mem Fund Q 56:297, 1968.
59. Djukanovic V, Mach EP (eds): Alternative Approaches to Meeting Basic Health Needs in Developing Countries. Geneva, WHO, 1975.
60. Sidel VW, Sidel R: Serve the People. New York, Josiah Macy Foundation, 1973.
61. Tang RCP: Community efforts in the delivery of health services in Hong Kong. In McNeur RW (ed): The Changing Roles and Education of Health Personnel Worldwide in View of the Increase of Basic Health Services. Philadelphia, Society for Health and Human Values, 1978, pp 167–184.
62. McKnight JL: Community health in a Chicago slum. Development Dialogue 1:62, 1978.
63. Guest I: Preventing heart disease through community action: the North Karelia Project. Development Dialogue 1:51, 1978.

CHAPTER 2

COMMUNITY DIAGNOSIS AND HEALTH SURVEILLANCE IN PRIMARY HEALTH CARE

The field of community health care requires epidemiologic foundations for action whether in large or small population groups. Diagnosis of the state of health of a community is as important for community health care as is careful diagnosis of the state of health of an individual patient seeking care.[1-5] If such diagnostic foundations are to be laid for action and treatment programs, the special personnel and tools required must be built into community health practice. A modern hospital could not function without special investigative manpower, laboratories, and other diagnostic facilities, which are essential for diagnosis and evaluation of change in patients' health. Community-oriented primary health care requires the same kinds of experts, as well as others trained in community diagnosis, such as epidemiologists, biostatisticians, and social scientists, with their equipment and laboratories.

There is need for much further study into ways of carrying out community diagnosis and health surveillance as an integral part of primary health care. Is there a value in such studies? The answer can come only from research into the uses of community diagnosis in primary health care.

The basic elements of community diagnosis include investigation of the community's state of health and its determinants. Community diagnosis should be seen as a continuing process along with planning, decision making, and action programs aimed to promote health of the community, prevent disease, treat the sick, and rehabilitate the disabled. As an ongoing process, it includes measures that also monitor health. Thus, mortality and morbidity trends are both diagnostic of the state of health of a community and, at the same time, a means of continuing health surveillance of that community. This is important in deciding on the data to be gathered, stored, and retrieved for analysis. Another important implication of this approach to diagnosis and surveillance as a unified ongoing process is that diagnosis does not necessarily precede action. It accompanies it.

Community diagnosis must become an integral part of primary health care if such care is to expand to include community health as well as care of individual patients. It is one of the important uses of epidemiology. Describing the state of health of a population and finding causes for the differential distribution of health conditions in different population groups is a function of epidemiology. Special consideration needs to be given to the use of epidemiology in community diagnosis and health surveillance of the small populations in primary health care practices.

COMMUNITY HEALTH AND ITS DETERMINANTS

Regarding health as a state of well-being and not merely the absence of disease is essential if community-oriented primary health care is to have promotive, preventive, alleviative, curative, and rehabilitative functions. The definition of health should include health-relevant characteristics such as somatic, psychologic, behavioral, and social, as well as an internationally recognized classification of disease, injuries, and causes of death. It should also take cognizance of the perceptions of health of the particular community.

Like that of an individual, a community's health reflects the interaction of its inheritance, environment, and life experience. The inheritance of a community is both genetic and cultural, which together with various attributes of the environment determine the life experience of all in the community. The totality of life experiences of each individual is unique to that person, but much of it is shared with others in the community and its subgroups. It is the process of internalization that makes a "happening" into a life experience, and this ongoing process of internalization of life experiences continually modifies the phenotype of each person in the community. Well-being and disease are attributes of the phenotype, which are manifested in somatic, psychologic, social, or behavioral characteristics of relevance to health (Fig. 2-1).

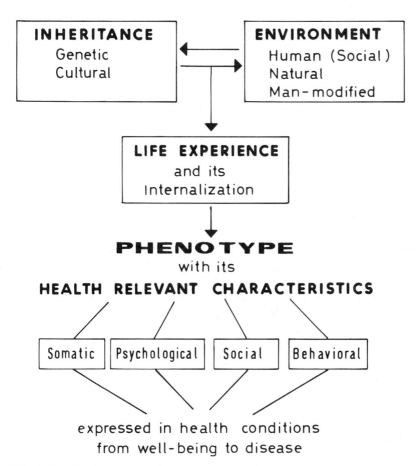

FIG. 2-1.   Health and its determinants—a diagrammatic representation.

Well-Being and Health

Well-being as such is seldom assessed in health care. The promotion and preservation of health have made little headway as a central interest of medicine, and hence health supervision has played an insignificant part in the diagnostic scheme of the primary-care physician. Its development has been in separate maternal and child health centers, in school health and occupational health services. However, even in these services the emphasis in diagnosis is on early detection of disease or screening of those who are at high risk for subsequent development of disease.

The concept of well-being, or healthiness, includes the subjective feeling of well-being, soundness of body and mind, and social functioning consistent with expected roles in society.

Among the pioneer ventures in assessing the state of well-being and health of a population was that of Williamson and Pearse in their Peckham experiment.[6-8] Their concept of health was something different from disease, and, therefore, they believed that the practice of health should differ from medicine, which was concerned with disease. Their early experience had shown that there were three categories of people, those in whom disorder was accompanied by "dis-ease," those in whom it was masked by compensation and who therefore felt themselves to be in a state of well-being, and lastly those in whom no disorder, disease, or disability was detected. This last group they called the "healthy." They designed and built a health center, which was a family and community club designed for the leisure activities of 2000 families. The objectives were to promote health of the families through a health center with a wide range of activities, including swimming in the indoor pool, gymnastics, badminton, table tennis, cricket net practice, billiards, skating, dancing, and other games such as chess, draughts, and cards.

Periodic health examinations and observations of members in their activities provided the basis for an appraisal of biologic and social health. Today, almost a half-century later, the Peckham approach remains a distinctive contribution, perhaps too different to survive in contemporary society, which perceives health as merely the absence or containment of disease.

While well-being is seldom diagnosed, emphasis on health as an attribute having a wider meaning than the absence of disease is written into the constitution of the World Health Organization, which states that health is "a state of complete physical, mental, and social well-being and not merely the absence of disease or infirmity."[9] This concept may yet have an influence on primary health care. Efforts to define and measure this elusive quality continue. These include studies of the congruence between sense of well-being, a subjective psychologic phenomenon, with more objective clinical and performance observations.[10]

As expected, various findings indicate that physical disorders exert an increasing influence on the feeling of well-being with increase in age. In a study of the elderly, physician and individual self-rating of health were found to be congruent over time, but more important was that the individual's self-rating was more predictive of later physician's rating than vice versa.[11]

Developmental examinations of infants and children are in fact measurements of health. These include a number of qualities: motor development, adaptive behavior with development of skills, personal-social behavior, and language. Similarly, intelligence tests and school performance are measures of "educational" functioning and subsequent social and economic abilities. The fact that performance of a number of socially relevant functions is included in the concept of well-being or health introduces culture-determined values and behavior. Thus, health will be measured according to different criteria in various culture groups, including communities, ethnic groups, and social classes. In cross-cultural comparisons and inferences, careful attention should be given to this, especially in mental and social health appraisal and self-perception of health.

Despite the general lack of advance in diagnosis of well-being, there is progress toward an integration of surveillance of health of children with their general medical care. There have been proposals for the special training of general practitioners to enable them to carry out the preventive aspects of child health care, including surveillance of child development.[12] Reports are also being published of the results of programs in which all children under 5 are included in a program of developmental surveillance in a general practice.[13]

Disease and Disability

Describing the distribution of disease and disability in a community requires a system of classification, in which various diseases and disabilities may be grouped according to an agreed convention. Diseases differ in the main systems they affect, in their clinical expression, and in their causes. Thus, while we need to use standardized criteria for their classification as well as similar or comparable methods of examination, the complexity of the problem of a universally satisfactory classification is well recognized. A system that is suitable for classifying causes of death may not be satisfactory for describing hospitalized cases, and neither of these is likely to meet the needs of describing disease and disability in community-based primary health care. Nevertheless, it is worthwhile to continue to seek and test a system that would provide a common basis for these varied uses.

Disease, injury, or other cause of morbidity are so commonly associated with varying degrees of disability that disease classification by itself is not sufficient as an indicator of illness in a community. This is especially so for purposes of community-oriented primary health care in an aging population, or any community in which chronic disease is common and where numbers of patients require home care as a result of being housebound. Therefore, an associated classification of diseases and disability is needed. Interference with expected role performance, inability to carry out activities of daily living, and limitation in mobility are among the indices of disability associated with disease. The extent of the disability is not always associated with the severity of the main disease diagnosed. The fact that the disease alone does not explain the extent of disability reinforces the case for widening various classifications of disease to include functional capacity and disability indices in primary-care practice concerned with communities.

There are various measures of disability in use. The National Center for Health Statistics of the United States has used simple definitions of limitation of mobility and major activities.[14] A number of indices have also been used for measuring activities of daily living (ADL).[15,16] These have been reviewed elsewhere.[5]

The most recent proposals for the international classification of diseases, the ninth revision published by the World Health Organization in 1977, outlines the history of development of such a universal system, from the original listing of causes of death well over a century ago through to its application to nonfatal cases and hospital recording systems, and to its present use in the evaluation of medical care.[17] This advance toward greater refinement and detail is taking place at the same time as there is increasing appreciation of the need to develop special classification systems for use in primary health care.[18]

Of special interest is the considerable extension of a supplementary classification of factors influencing health status and contact with health services.[17] This classification includes provision for persons who have contact with health services for reasons other than illness or injury. Provision is made for people exposed to potential health hazards, such as exposure to communicable disease, the need for immunization, isolation, or other prophylactic measures, and personal or family history of various diseases and allergies. It also provides for classification of persons having contact with health services for purposes related to reproduction, such as contraception, care during pregnancy and the puerperium, and during growth and development through infancy and childhood. It also includes contacts for administrative purposes, such as the issue of medical certificates; and a number of conditions influencing health, such as problems with vision, and other special functions; and a variety of socioeconomic and family conditions, such as housing, unemployment, and other deprivations. Of importance in community-oriented primary care is the provision for recording contacts with individuals for investigations including screening examinations and population surveys.

The Community Syndrome Concept

The concept of a clinical syndrome is central to clinical diagnosis, which involves a process of eliciting a number of related symptoms and signs. When these occur together in a cluster, they are suggestive of a clinical syndrome that constitutes a particular disease. The syndrome may be caused by a single underlying pathologic process, but often it is a product of several processes which, interacting with one another, produce a final common expression.

Community diagnosis similarly involves finding an association between various states of health in a community. The prevention of disease is often focused on action that will effect the occurrence of a group of diseases. The diseases may be transmitted by a common vehicle, such as water. Among the best recognized of these are the diarrheal diseases, each with its own immediate microbiologic cause that can be prevented by such action as improved water supplies and food hygiene. Similarly, the prevention of diseases of malnutrition is not necessarily best done by the use of specific nutrients, but rather by a modified balanced diet containing the specific deficient nutrients. The concept of balance is important in such preventive work, imbalance being accompanied by exacerbation of various elements of nutritional failure syndromes.

The concept of a community syndrome involves several considerations. First, there is the association in occurrence of a number of health conditions. This co-prevalence or co-incidence may include various diseases, as well as somatic, psychosocial, or behavioral characteristics. However, a community syndrome is more than the association of a number of diseases and health characteristics. It is their interaction that constitutes the essence of the concept. Thus, co-prevalence and interaction are central elements of it. As indicated, a community syndrome may result from different causes, each having its effects on a particular element of the syndrome. On the other hand, the determinants or causes, like the health syndrome itself, may constitute an interacting network of factors, which together produce the syndrome. For practical purposes, investigation of community syndromes can be built around common and important disorders in the particular community. This applies especially to diseases that may be better prevented, or treated, if recognized in the context of the epidemiologically defined syndrome of which they are a part. Diagrammatic representations of two community syndromes are presented here. Figure 2-2 represents a community syndrome of poverty, malnutrition, infectious diseases, and "possession" in a peasant community. Figure 2-3 shows a community syndrome of coronary heart disease in

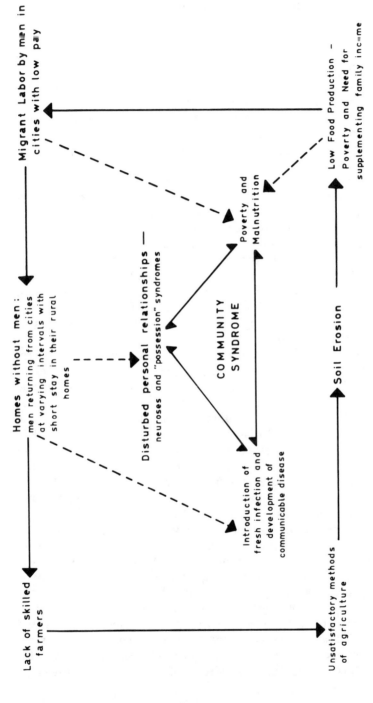

FIG. 2-2. Community syndrome of poverty, malnutrition, infectious disease, and "possession." [From Kark, 1974 (see Ref. 5).]

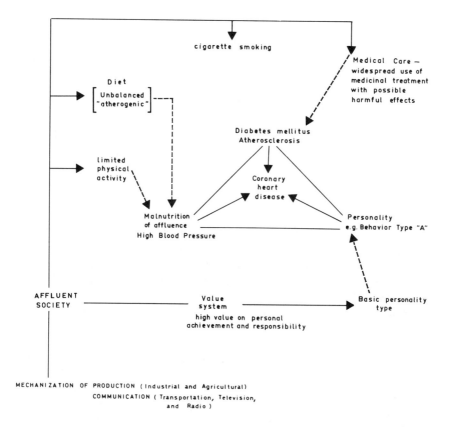

FIG. 2-3. Community syndrome of coronary heart disease. [From Kark, 1974 (see Ref. 5).]

more affluent communities with their nutritional imbalance and excesses, drive for achievement, and other personality characteristics.

Life Experience and the Environment

At conception, a newly formed zygote inherits a constitution and begins activity as a new individual interacting with its environment. This is the beginning of a continuing life experience of the individual in the environment. The meaningful element of life experience is that which has been internalized and thereby becomes an integral part of the individual (Fig. 2-1). The life experience of individuals determines, and is itself determined by, their growth and development. Each phase of growth is succeeded by the next in a genetically ordered pattern characteristic for the species. Therefore, the kind of development during one phase may be expected to influence succeeding phases, and the effects of different experiences on growth will depend on the phases of development at which they happen. Thus, understanding congenital malformations requires knowledge of events and experiences that have distinct effects at different developmental phases of the fetus, such as maternal rubella. Similarly, widely differing kinds of life experiences may be expected to affect individuals differently according to the phase of life at which they occur. This would include such processes as immunologic responses to different antigens, the nutritional and metabolic effects of various diets, mental development, and personal-social functioning in response to varied learning experiences in groups, such as the family and other small, intimate primary groups.

Life experience is an active process of interaction between individuals and their environments, with developmental changes producing a succession of phenotypes. The health-relevant characteristics of the phenotype are its biologic, psychologic, behavioral, and social qualities. The environmental characteristics of special relevance to health of a communty are the social, physical, and biologic.

The Social Environment.   The social or human environment includes consideration of aspects of the social system, human relationships, culture, and economic state.

The quality of the relationship network within which individuals are reared and function throughout their lives is central to any concept of health. In fact, it is social health. Essential for health are supportive, affectional one-to-one relationships, such as those of a loving, accepting mother and her baby,[19] the reciprocal support of confidants,[20] or the love of a mate[21]; the solidary and affectional relationships within a small group, family, or friends; and the sense of belonging, and of stability, associated with being part of a community in social equilibrium as opposed to anomie.[22-25] While each of these relational groups warrants further study in its implications for health, sufficient is now understood for them to be of importance in primary health care. The life experience of individuals is determined by the family and community into which they are born; its customs mold their habits, and its beliefs and values become theirs; they become an integral part of its network of relationships; its social status or class is their initial ascribed status; its educational and economic level is a determinant of the physique, nutrition, and material well-being of its members.

The transmission of culture is a social heritage shared by members of that culture; as such, it is a force making for social stability and equilibrium. Equally characteristic of society are social, economic, and cultural changes. These changes have a profound impact on health, the disease patterns of different societies, secular trends in the growth of children, the physique of men and women, and probably on the personality types prevalent in different groups.

Of relevance to community health and health care are different qualities of society, which range from extremes of stability and change, equilibrium and disequilibrium, conflict and harmony, affluence and poverty. Not only is the social system an important determinant of health and disease, but the interaction between genotype and the varied elements of the natural environment is moderated by social and cultural factors. The macroclimate is modified by the community in its clothing and housing, the reconstruction of waterways, and numerous other artifacts. No less important than these material considerations, and in fact underlying many of them, are people's perceptions of their environment. Health professionals working in settings in which the prevailing beliefs and concepts about the environment are very different from their own require understanding of, knowledge about, and sensitivity to cultural differences. It is important to stress that this is applicable in all situations in which the community and health professionals are not culturally homogeneous. This involves consideration of differences such as those of education, socioeconomic status, ethnic and religious affiliations.

Studies of different cultures by anthropologists, and of changing societies by social historians, illustrate this capacity to understand other peoples' perceptions of the world around them. Learning to think like the people of communities whose health one seeks to improve was a basic objective of Benjamin Paul's pioneer symposium on health, culture, and community.[26]

Among the important implications of culture for health are customs, value orientations, and belief systems.

Customs.   Health-relevant examples of customary practices are:

Diet, smoking, alcohol, and drug abuse.
Personal hygiene and cleanliness of the immediate environs.
Role functioning according to age and sex in work, play, school, and family.
Sex and mating, marriage, family formation and spacing, contraceptive practices.
Infant and child-rearing practices.
Modern and traditional health care systems and their use.

Value Orientations and Belief Systems.   Value attitudes of a community vary for the sexes, different age groups, social classes, and religious groups. Those of health relevance include different moral standards, constraints, socially acceptable behavior, and religious health practices.

Belief systems of a community extend through such areas as its health knowledge and medical practices, from beliefs in witchcraft to the influence of social environment on health, and from "possession" by demons and evil spirits to the germ theory.

There are also different beliefs about the influence of various foodstuffs on health and behavior, traditional medicinal herbs and mixtures, and more modern beliefs in pills and injections.

The Physical and Biologic Environment.   The natural environment and its modification by man is the other aspect of environment that is of importance to health. Adaptation to environment is a process of natural selection, culturally and biologically determined responses to the vagaries of climate, vegetation, and fauna. Perhaps the most dramatic impacts of natural environment on health are periodic disasters, caused by cyclones, floods, earthquakes, and volcanic eruptions.

Among the influences of natural environment of interest in the setting of primary health care are the climatic rhythms, such as the seasonal occurrence of various diseases, and the circadian rhythm of physiologic variables such as blood pressure. Microbacteria, viruses, and vectors of various pathogenic organisms, and the diseases they spread through vast areas of the world, are perhaps the most studied aspects of natural environment in medicine and public health. Hence, they will be of considerable concern to primary health care. In fact, however, public health control measures of these diseases have tended to exclude the primary-care network of services. In this way, a major instrument of potential benefit has not been effectively used. The widespread occurrence of diseases due to insanitary conditions, such as gastroenteritis in infants, is indicative of the need for attention to the most basic forms of sanitary disposal of human excreta and the protection of food and water. The villagers and peasants of the world, and the masses of rural migrants pouring into the rapidly growing city slums, are exposed to infections that are readily controlled by health services oriented toward such community needs.

While the long-term approach to diarrheal diseases involves improvements in nutrition, water supplies, and food hygiene, simple methods of oral rehydration therapy prevent, or effectively treat, their major cause of serious illness and death, dehydration. The public health programs for improved nutrition and water supplies should therefore be linked with primary-care facilities, as recommended by WHO and UNICEF.[27]

Man-modified or man-made environmental conditions have much of interest for community-oriented primary health care, including pollution of air, water, soil, and food by unsatisfactory disposal of excreta, refuse, and various wastes from homes and industry. Industrialization, and the technologic advances that have made it possible, have enabled people to live in larger and more densely concentrated crowded cities. Hazards to community health increase not only with the spread of industry, but also with the widening of industrial processes. Accidents, exposure to industrial dusts and chemicals, noise, or radiation, and other conditions of work, crowding, lack of leisure time, and pressure, all add to the challenge that faces a considerable segment of present-day urban societies. This has important implications for community-oriented primary health care, including services based in factories and other places of work.

Locality. This is perhaps the most important environmental consideration in community-oriented primary health care. Differences in the health of people living in different localities are well known, and have been reported for such widely differing disorders as juvenile delinquency and crime on the one hand and infant mortality, tuberculosis, and mental disorder on the other.[28] Locality of residence in cities is determined by social and economic factors and is itself a marker of social differentiation and stratification. The social class structure of a city tends to express itself in a distinctive geographic distribution of the different classes in the city. Working-class neighborhoods, slums and poverty quarters, middle- and upper-middle class, and ethnic group areas are often to be found in separated, relatively well-demarcated parts of the city. It is thus to be expected that there will be marked differences in major demographic and social characteristics, in the physical environment, and in the health states of the various groups served by different primary health care practices.

The differentiation between areas is evident in growing cities and was well illustrated in the pioneer ecologic studies of the American city reported earlier in this century by Park and Burgess.[29,30] The distinctive social class, ethnic, or nativity characteristics of neighborhoods, streets, or wider localities of residence are a feature of present-day city living. Big metropolitan cities, such as New York and London, have considerable areas of the inner city inhabited by large numbers of immigrants from more rural areas of the country or from foreign countries. The influence of locality on primary health care goes beyond the different disease patterns of the communities to differences in use of services and participation in local neighborhood development.

Measurement of Characteristics of the Community and Its Environment

Community-oriented primary health care needs to be selective in its approach to community diagnosis and in determining priorities for action, since effort, time, and cost are required for gathering, analyzing, interpreting, and evaluating the data.

Community diagnosis in primary health care is more readily carried out in the framework of care provided to a defined population. The population may be defined by membership or by registration, by geographic area of residence, or by place of work. The service may be provided from a neighborhood health center, a group practice, a factory or student clinic, or other primary-care facilities. Large and crowded inner-city populations offer a considerable challenge to the organization of community-oriented primary health care, more especially in defining the population. In rural communities and small towns, gathering the data required for community diagnosis may be easier, since the population is more readily defined.

Making a community diagnosis, and maintaining a system of surveillance of the community's changing state of health, involves the systematic collection of data about the community, its environment, and various facets of its health. The emphasis will depend on the priority given to various conditions by the community and the primary health care team. This will depend on the kind of community, its social, economic, and cultural characteristics, locality, and housing conditions. They are as varied as are the individuals who live in them, including middle-class residential neighborhoods and suburban communities of the city, new housing projects in high-rise buildings, peripheral slums, and deteriorating inner-city zones, small towns and farming communities, poor peasant communities, isolated fishing villages, and migrant populations.

How does one systematize community diagnosis under such widely differing circumstances? One wonders that it has not yet been done, only to realize that the demand or know-how has not been there. Community-oriented primary health care is not yet developed as a feature of health and medical services, and yet for those of us who consider this approach essential for adequate health care, it must be attempted. This involves data collection of health and disease conditions and their determinants in the community in order to make a community diagnosis, on the basis of which action can be taken and the effects evaluated.

The Community: Demographic and Social Data

The traditional primary-care practitioner of Western societies, the family or village doctor, was renowned for his knowledge about the people he doctored. It was wisdom born of the experience in his day-to-day practice and his own participation in the activities of the social world of which he was a part. However, this does not meet the present-day needs of community-oriented primary health care. Helpful as it may be in giving a subjective picture of the community and its main health problems, the systematic development of demographic and other relevant data is essential for community diagnosis in primary care.

It is usual to describe the health of a community by comparing various health indices of groups within the community itself and those of other populations. The use of variables defining different groups of a community changes according to the kind of community and the particular health condition being measured. There are demographic characteristics of universal usefulness in differentiating between groups in a community. These include basic biologic characteristics such as age and sex, social categories such as social status and role, and biosocial characteristics such as family and ethnic groups. A community health center or a group practice clinic will therefore require a record system that will include information on the community eligible to use the service. The minimal inclusions in such a register are age and sex, occupation, education, family, kinship and ethnic group, religion, social class or socioeconomic status, locality, and migration.

Age and Sex.   All individuals in the practice should be registered according to their sex and date of birth, by a recording system that makes these data readily available for analysis of various community health indices and changes in the age and sex structure of the community.

The main health indices of interest in primary health care are incidence and prevalence rates of various diseases in different age groups according to sex, or age-specific rates. When comparing the frequency of disease in the population served by a particular primary health center, or group practice, with that of other populations, it is important to appreciate that the age distribution of the populations may be different. Allowance is made for this by adjustment or standardization for age, the methods for which are available in many texts of public health statistics.

Another index of interest is the male : female ratio of various disorders, and the changes that may occur over time. Again, such comparisons need to be based on age-specific rates in the two sexes, or on age-adjusted rates.

Occupation. The register should show the occupation of all individuals in two ways. First, details of the person's occupation, and second, the classification of the occupations by social class or socioeconomic status, using an accepted method.

Education. The simplest way of recording education is to enter details of the highest educational achievement, taking into consideration all education, including regular schools, professional schools, technical and religious institutions. This should then be summarized by a figure representing the total years of formal education, for example, 0, 8, 12, 20 years.

Family. A number of family indices may be used in community diagnosis. These include marital status, maternal history, and structure and size of the family. These, and other relevant details, are best recorded on a household or family health census.

Kinship. Detailed genealogic charts, or family trees, are of special interest in certain genetic or other health conditions having a familial aggregation. There are also some communities in which kinship networks are an outstanding feature of the social structure, and thus may have health implications of interest to primary-care practitioners.

Ethnic Group. As in the family kinship unit, an ethnic group has both biologic and social features of health importance. A common method of ethnic classification is by country of origin, since such groups often share a distinctive cultural tradition and ancestry. They may thus have genetic characteristics, as well as shared habits, values, or religious beliefs of importance to their health.

Religion. The interest of religion for community-oriented primary health care goes beyond the analysis of health conditions according to stated religion. In certain communities, religiosity should also be noted, as religious conviction and practice, rather than nominal religious affiliation, may have a profound influence on health and behavior of relevance to health.[21,31,32] Thus, one may note a scale from orthodox to nonreligious, such as: devout, orthodox, strict adherence to religious precepts and practices; occasional participation in religious services, or the performance of some traditional religious practices; nonpracticing or secular.

Social Class or Socioeconomic Status.[33,34] Various operational definitions of social class have been used in epidemiologic studies of health and health care.[5] The commonest methods involve ranking from upper to lower classes. Ranking by occupation is the foundation of the well-known systems used by the United States Census[35] and by the British registrar-general.[36,37] Others have combined several variables—occupation, education, and neighborhood of residence—giving different weighting to each.[38] For international use in European countries, Brichler suggested a classification by social and economic characteristics that does not include a ranking system.[39]

Locality.   Among the physical features that differentiate residential areas are the following health-relevant characteristics:

> The material, maintenance, and development of housing, its spatial distribution ranging from high-rise apartment buildings to single-family houses set in their own gardens.
>
> Development of roads, sidewalks, and parks with provision for flow of traffic and parking facilities, play centers for children, sport and leisure-time facilities.
>
> Shopping areas and other amenities, community centers, schools, health and welfare service buildings, their proximity and accessibility.
>
> Water supplies, lighting of houses and streets, systems of disposal of waste and excreta.
>
> Standard of cleanliness of neighborhood, including absence of garbage litter.

The People in the Neighborhood.   In addition to the personal characteristics listed earlier, observations on personal appearance, clothing, and activities are useful.

The stability of residence and community services are of health relevance, and in some areas measurement of migration, in and outward movements, are a central feature of the health picture.

Measurement of Community Health

Making a community diagnosis is a process involving the collection of information over time, thus building a data base from which an increasing number of health indices may be calculated. Gathering the data required to build up knowledge for community diagnosis not only takes time, but should be done gradually on the basis of priorities. Some of it may be done by special surveys, but much of the information can be included routinely on family and individual clinical records. Furthermore, the records should be planned to allow for abstraction of data for epidemiologic as well as clinical purposes.

There are various ways of gathering data in a primary-care practice:

> Information from official and other agencies, such as data from a maternity hospital on a mother and her newborn baby; birth information from a government health office, which might include birth weight, length of gestation, and other data of relevance for health care; information on a patient discharged from hospital.

> Information from a service especially established for the screening of disease, such as a tuberculosis screening service, vision and hearing surveys.

> Special health examinations, such as measurement for blood pressure, hemoglobin, and weight, on people who usually turn to the doctor or nurse or who are registered for care with the practice. This can be done by inviting the individuals concerned to a special session arranged for the purpose, or by conducting the examinations on all patients at the time of their attending the practice.

The subject matter of special surveys will obviously depend on their purpose, such as identifying the main health problems of the community or periodically reviewing change in the community's health. Here, distinction should be made between health surveys or screening conducted in the framework of primary care and national health surveys or mass screening for a particular disease.

The purpose of a screening survey is essentially case finding. Mass screening surveys were initiated many years ago as part of the growing public health movement.[40] These specific surveys have included various procedures for detecting cases of disease or for surveillance of infection and its transmission. Among the important diseases included in such mass screening surveys have been tuberculosis, yaws, syphilis, leprosy, trachoma, and malaria. More recently, screening has extended to include other conditions, such as cancer of the breast, cancer of the cervix, or hypertension, and multiple screening procedures have also been developed. While the immediate objective is the detection of cases, screening may also be used for purposes of community diagnosis. This can best be developed if the initial planning and extension of the program includes epidemiologic methods and objectives.

Even when conducting a special survey, the gathering of information by a primary health care team is a different process from that of mass screening. The relatively familiar and personal nature of the contact is in marked contrast to the impersonal relationship and conduct of mass screening surveys. The response of the community may be expected to be different, especially in the compliance of those found to be in need of treatment. Despite these differences, some criteria are applicable to all forms of community health survey. The World Health Organization and various workers have outlined criteria that need to be met by screening tests if such surveys are to be ethical and effective.[41-46] While the subject has become prominent as a result of the increase in mass screening surveys, it is also relevant in the consideration of well-established procedures in general periodic health examinations, as well as examinations through pregnancy, infancy, and childhood. It thus warrants wider consideration, and the following is a summary of the criteria that should be met by any routine examination used to assess the state of health of individuals in their own interests or to make a community diagnosis.

Concerning the State of Health. *Screening for Disease.* The disease should be common or sufficiently serious to warrant a survey for screening of cases or for community diagnosis. The health team and the community should be interested in reducing its prevalence, preventing its incidence through action focused on the determinants, or at least assuring that cases are adequately treated. Thus, the disease itself should be known to be responsive to treatment; early diagnosis, and hence early treatment or behavior change, should improve the prognosis of affected cases and change the incidence and prevalence rates in the community. This last has special relevance when risk factors or other determinants of the disease are included in the survey.

Other Surveys of Health Status. Differing from surveys for screening cases of disease are those in which the primary objective is assessment of aspects of the community's health, such as child growth and nutritional state. Various anthropometric measurements, height, weight, skinfold thickness, and indices derived from them, such as the Quetelet index and the Ponderal index, are well established as indicators of nutritional status in certain circumstances.[47] Their use for initial commuity diagnosis, and subsequent periodic repeat examination for purposes of surveillance and evaluation of effectiveness of action, is only justifiable if the data are analyzed for these purposes.

The same principles apply to other health surveys of this kind, especially those in which measurement data of a single variable, or a group of variables, are used for appraisal of the state of health of a population group.

Concerning the Examination Procedures and Tests. While the examinations should be simple, they must have high reliability, and when used to screen for disease, must have high sensitivity and specificity. It is desirable that they should have been subjected to critical investigation in controlled clinical trials and that the results of these trials should be available to the primary health care team, who use the various tests as part of their routine examinations.

The costs of the test should warrant the information provided for community diagnosis and for screening of cases. This last aspect extends to the cost of treatment which, in turn, should be considered in relation to the importance of the disease.

Concerning the Community. The procedures involved in carrying out health examinations, or obtaining specimens for laboratory examination, should be simple and acceptable to members of the community. The individual, family, or community actions required should be ensured by sound relationships between the health team and the population. Community involvement and interest in the program should become an important feature of such surveys.

Whether the information is obtained from the practice itself or from other sources, the purposes of such surveys are usually to separate out those who have the condition from those who do not. In this respect it is an extension of case-finding measures to initiate care. However, they may have additional functions important for community-oriented primary care. Suitably planned, the information may be analyzed to provide knowledge on the prevalence of various conditions in the community. Measurement data, such as blood pressure, relative weight, and the findings of various laboratory examinations, can be analyzed in terms of frequency distributions, means or medians, and standard deviations. Both prevalence rates of disease or its risk factors and analysis of measurement data can be used for comparison between various groups within the community, or with other populations.

The data gathered in community health surveys need to be carefully considered. One cannot stress enough the importance of gathering and recording only those data that will be used. Computer printouts litter many offices, often stacked high in corners and on shelves; their information, although of much potential interest, is not used by the practice. Reasons could be that there is insufficient time or manpower, or that interest and enthusiasm may have diminished in the interval between collection and analysis of the data.

DECIDING ON PRIORITIES FOR COMMUNITY PROGRAMS IN PRIMARY HEALTH CARE

Community medicine programs in primary health care may be focused on different phases of the life span of individuals and families, as well as on the main health problems in the community. The ways in which the health team considers the priorities for community health care will determine the orientation of community diagnosis and health surveillance.

In a primary health care practice that provides promotive, preventive, and curative services, it is useful to focus on major developmental phases and social groups within the community. These include:

Reproduction and family formation.
Childhood, from infancy through adolescence to maturity.
Adulthood, aging, and the elderly.

Reproduction and Family Formation

Reproduction.   Two important measures of reproduction of interest in primary health care practice involving family and community health are the live-birth rate and the total fertility rate:

Live-Birth Rate: The number of live births in a year per 1000 persons in the average population of the community for that year.

Total Fertility Rate: The number of live births in a year per 1000 women aged 15 to 44 in the community.

Additional indices of interest in special circumstances are:

Age-specific fertility rates.
Age distribution of mothers, especially teenage (15 to 19) and older mothers (35 to 44 and over).
Reproduction rates, gross and net, may be of interest in primary health care to larger populations.

Family Formation. *Mating and Marriage.* Common questions of interest to couples include fertility control, sterility, advice regarding family size, genetic problems, and sex relationships. At this time, family spacing is perhaps the outstanding concern of health, welfare, and population authorities, as well as of a growing proportion of the community itself. While special contraceptive and family planning clinics have been established in many places, this is also a proper function of primary health care. It includes advice on family spacing and its meaning for family health, as well as contraceptive management and the implications of different contraceptives for health.

Family Information. The data required on the family include the following:

> Marital status of couple: married, never married, widowed, divorced, or separated, previous unions.
> One-parent family: married, separated, divorced, widowed, never married.
> Age at marriage of mother and father.
> Maternal history: age of mother at first pregnancy and birth of first child, history of pregnancies and outcome, including intervals between pregnancies.
> Family size: number of live births, number of surviving children, spacing between live births, desired number of children.
> Family structure: nuclear family, extended family, aged dependent member, living alone.
> Family status and other health-relevant variables: occupation and education of parents, other indicators of social status, with special reference to the particular community.
> Family relationships.
> Family problems: economic, housing, chronic illness, and disability.

Contraception. The data required include information on knowledge, attitudes, and practices in the community, and measures of the health services activities. For these purposes, population surveys may be made and have usually been planned as research studies rather than as an integral part of a community program conducted in the framework of primary health care. However, this can readily be done based on methods developed in research studies, but adapted to the cultural traditions of different communities.[48]

The WHO's International Classification of Diseases (9th revision) makes provision for recording details of this aspect of health care.[17]

Pregnancy and Its Outcome.   Maternal health is a central function of primary health care. In some cities, care through pregnancy, delivery, and puerperium is carried out by obstetricians, but in most areas community-based primary-care practitioners, such as physicians, public health nurses, and midwives, or their substitutes, are responsible. In more developed countries, with few exceptions, a large proportion of mothers are delivered in the hospital, while their prenatal and postnatal care may be carried out in special mother and child health clinics or in more integrated primary health services.

The minimal information required for pregnancy and its outcome includes:

Demographic data: age, marital status, parity, education, occupation, social class, ethnic group, religion.

Pregnancy history: present pregnancy, wanted, planned, previous pregnancies and their outcome, intervals between pregnancies, abortions, stillbirths and live births, family spacing.

Somatic characteristics: mother's height, weight, and weight changes during pregnancy, blood pressure and hemoglobin changes during pregnancy, blood group ABO, Rh.

Behavior: alcohol, smoking, drug addiction, medications, diet.

Progress of the pregnancy: normal pregnancy, morbidity mainly related to pregnancy, and general morbidity during pregnancy, such as diabetes, heart disease, psychiatric disorder.

Fetal health and growth: prenatal screening, procedures for detection of fetal abnormality and growth retardation.

Outcome of pregnancy: normal live-born infant and type of birth, birth weight, period of gestation, abortive outcome, stillbirth, congenital anomalies.

Delivery and labor: normal labor and delivery, complications, and methods of delivery.

Puerperium: normal, complications of the puerperium.

Postpartum care and examination.

Perinatal period (fetal age 28 weeks to newborn through first week): normal, abnormal conditions originating in the perinatal period, perinatal mortality.

Childhood and Adolescence

The health state of the child population of a community may be best assessed in different age and sex groups; the grouping will depend on the particular community. In more developed countries, children attend school for a considerable period of their childhood, and it is suggested that this period, which separates early childhood from late adolescence, is the natural division for practical purposes of community health care. We thus have three main groups:

Infancy and preschool age childhood (birth to 4 years).

School age children (5 to 18 years, and maybe less in particular countries).

Postschool age to adulthood (18 or younger, up to 20 years). This is of special importance in communities in which children leave school at younger ages.

Community diagnosis should help define the major health problems in these three main groups of the child population by defining their health characteristics in terms of relevant physical, psychologic, behavioral, and social variables, as well as morbidity, accidental injury, disability, and mortality.

Infancy and Preschool Childhood (the Under-Fives).   The health of an infant at birth is a product of its genetic constitution, prenatal life experience, and the birth process itself. Records on birth status should therefore include information on these factors.

The main determinants of health through infancy are nutrition, mothering and loving care, protection from injury, harmful agents or infection.

Infant Mortality Rates.   Among the main indices of infant health are various mortality rates, namely, the perinatal, neonatal, postneonatal, and total infant mortality. The commonly used infant mortality rates are:

Infant mortality rate (IMR): The number of deaths in the first year of life per 1000 live births in a year.

Neonatal mortality rate: The number of deaths in infants under 28 days of age per 1000 live births in a year.

Perinatal mortality rate: The number of deaths from 28 weeks fetal life through to first week of life per 1000 live births in a year.

In many more developed countries, there has been a considerable decline in these rates, beginning with a reduction in postneonatal deaths, especially from causes such as gastroenteritis and pneumonia, then during the later weeks of the neonatal period, and more recently a fall in perinatal mortality rate.

In countries with low infant mortality rates, these may not be discriminating indices in the relatively small populations usually served by primary health care centers. However, registers of deaths may be maintained by such units, with reviews by the health team of their causes, preventability, the care provided prior to death, and implications for the family of such a crisis.

In less developed countries infant mortality rates are generally much higher. A main problem is that of obtaining and recording information on births and deaths of infants. Primary health care teams often need to introduce their own system of registration for this purpose.

Morbidity. In infancy, especially postneonatal (from age 4 weeks to 1 year), gastroenteritis and acute respiratory illnesses are common, and are often serious, being the main causes of hospitalization of infants. Hospitalizations for these illnesses, as well as their diagnosis in primary care, can be readily recorded. The rates of these conditions are especially useful in those centers serving a defined population and used as the major primary-care service for children. Registers for all children with congenital malformations and genetic conditions, chronic disease and disabilities, psychologic and social handicaps need to be maintained.

As might be expected, the health of infants and young children in various communities differs considerably, and there are wide variations in mortality and morbidity rates, in growth and intellectual development, in health-relevant behavior and social pathology. The fact that a community is part of a large city and metropolitan area of a developed country does not ensure it a high standard of health, and differences in the state of health of different communities in the same city are well known. Thus, each population served by a particular primary-care facility needs study, and the findings should be related to the wider area in which the community is situated.

Growth and Development, and Their Determinants. As already indicated, some of the rates and indices of health that are applicable in large populations may not be so useful when the denominator is small, as in many primary-care health centers or general practices. However, a number of measurements, in addition to those for mortality and morbidity, are very useful and helpful in making a community diagnosis. Among these are:

> *Growth and development:*
> Physical, weight, length or height, skinfold thickness.
> Psychomotor, motor, adaptive, social, language development.
> Intelligence tests, specially designed for children of preschool ages.

Nutritional status:
Anthropometric measurements, clinical manifestations, and laboratory tests.

Health-relevant behavior:
The earliest measures include such data as various psychomotor tests, feeding, response to mother, and later, developmental and play activities.

Relationships:
Living with mother or substitute mother, marital status of mother, recognition by father, structure of family in which child lives, evidence of neglect, rejection, "battered baby."

School Age Children. *Mortality and Morbidity.* The diseases affecting the child population will vary considerably, but accidents are a major cause of disability and mortality.

Basic records should include all diagnoses and problems noted in children by the primary-care practice, at the clinic or health center, at home, and at school. In addition, the following health-relevant characteristics are of interest to primary health care of any community:

Somatic:
Growth, height, weight, nutrition status, maturation, hearing, vision, dental health, genetic markers relevant to community.

Psychologic:
Educational progress, Intelligence Quotient, personality and behavior, ability to relate with others.

Behavior:
Play, participation in sport and recreational activities.
Diet.
Sex behavior, contraception, teenage pregnancy.
Deviant behavior, absenteeism from school or work without acceptable causes, drug addiction, cigarette smoking, alcohol, various forms of delinquency.

Social:
Family background, social support, social participation and activities, religion and religious activities, postschool vocational and higher education, employment.

Disability:
Chronic or life-threatening diseases, physical, mental, and social handicaps.

Adulthood, Aging, and the Aged

We have considered some elements of adulthood, namely, mating and family formation. Much of the primary-care contact with adult women concerns their functions in reproduction, child-rearing, and family, including care of their aging parents. However, health care of women and men extends beyond these family functions, to include work and other activities. There may be primary-care facilities in their neighborhood of living, at their place of work, or they may use the ambulant care services of a major hospital. We are concerned here with the community- or work-based type of primary care, which are both communal and individual in their orientation.

Registers of mortality and morbidity should be maintained, including details of deaths in the community, chronic illness, and disability, and selected findings of well-being or disorder obtained from special surveys, such as preemployment examinations and periodic health examinations.

Should special surveys be made for common conditions such as hypertension, or should existing primary-care facilities undertake routine examinations of blood pressure of all patients, or at least all adult patients, attending for care? When primary-care facilities are readily accessible, a large proportion of the population has been found to use the service, and thus over a period of a relatively few years the vast majority might have their blood pressure measured.[49] There is also the question of cost. Case finding in general practice has been shown to be less costly than that of special screening clinics set up in the community.[50] Thus, if primary-care practitioners can be motivated to introduce such a routine for all who attend their practices, an important step would be taken in gathering the data needed to make the most elementary form of community diagnosis of the prevalence of hypertension, and the distribution of systolic and diastolic blood pressures, while identifying those who are likely to benefit by treatment.

The data gathered may extend beyond this. Thus, in communities in which coronary artery disease and diabetes mellitus are common, it is advisable to include the measurement of additional variables. This would allow for more sophisticated epidemiologic co-prevalence studies of a community syndrome of cardiovascular and metabolic diseases and their risk factors.

In addition, health-relevant characteristics of adults are of much interest in the type of community-oriented primary care being reviewed here. Much of the basic data is similar to that suggested for childhood and adolescence, the emphasis in the former being on growth to maturity, while in adulthood we are more concerned with health and disease during the years of maturity and aging. Among the health characteristics of interest, over and above mortality and recognized morbidity are:

Somatic:
Weight and height. Differences in height by age may suggest further investigation of secular change in growth.
Blood pressure, lipid levels, blood sugar and uric acid levels, hemoglobin.
Infection, nutritional status, dental health, genetic markers.

Psychologic:
Personality inventories, such as interviews or behavior schedules for "A" and "B" behavior types, Cattels' Personality Factor Test.
Special tests: memory, especially related to aging, intelligence.

Behavior:
Diet, emphasis will vary according to major health problems such as protein and calorie deficiency in poorer groups, sugar (sucrose) in all groups, fats, carbohydrates, and fibers.
Sex, exercise, smoking, alcohol and drug addiction, personal deviant behavior.

Social:
Social situation: family status, work, occupational and educational status, social participation.
Change: in employment, family status, migration. Sudden change or life crisis as in mass disasters, floods, earthquakes, war, or personal and family crisis, such as death or sudden illness of family member or close friend.

Family health history:
Parents and siblings of individuals. If alive, age and health condition; if deceased, age and cause of death.

INCIDENCE AND PREVALENCE RATES

The frequency of a disease or disability is most often expressed as a rate or ratio of those who have the condition and the total, or exposed, population. It is calculated as a rate per unit of population depending on convention or convenience (per 100; 1000; 10,000; 100,000). Two rates, incidence and prevalence, are in general use to describe the frequency of diseases.

Incidence.   The incidence rate of a disease measures the number of new cases that occur during a defined period of time in the population at risk, and is calculated as follows:

$$\frac{\text{Number of new cases of the disease during a particular period of time}}{\text{Population at that time (usually taken as the average population at risk during that time)}} \times 1000$$

Birth and death rates, and rates of events such as accidents and injuries, are also incidence rates.

Prevalence.   The prevalence rate of a disease or disability measures the total number of cases at a particular time in the population at that time, and may be expressed as follows:

$$\frac{\text{Number of cases of the disease at a particular time}}{\text{Population at that time}} \times 1000$$

Denominator Information.   For purposes of public health reporting on the health of populations, this information is usually derived from census data. However, this is not always possible in primary health care. The population served by a neighborhood health center, or by a primary-care practitioner, may not necessarily coincide with the population within the census tracts used for census purposes. In this respect, estimates from data in census tracts may sometimes be helpful. In many countries, families and individuals who are eligible to use a health facility are required to register with it, as in health insurance agencies, health maintenance organizations, and the British National Health Service.[51-53] In this service, members of the population select the doctor (general practitioner) of their choice, and the average list of a doctor is approximately 2000 persons. It is this registered population that would constitute the denominator. If there were five to ten doctors practicing from a health center, or in a group practice, the combined population would range between 10,000 and 25,000.

In crowded inner-city communities often populated by immigrants and poorer people, and in medically less developed countries, primary-care health centers may not so readily obtain detailed information on the population. However, with community health workers employed in increasing numbers in many countries, a household health census may be maintained by them for the population served by a primary health center. One approach to this difficult and important problem is described in more detail in Chapter 8. Much depends on the importance attached to the development of community medicine as an integral part of primary health care, and hence of the functions of the manpower employed in such services.

The kind and amount of denominator information and the way it is gathered and recorded will differ in various practices. Periodic updating of information is vital, for example, changes in health status, occupation, education, or family composition, through births, deaths, and migration. Wherever possible, the records should be similar to those of the population census and the main health records of the country. In this way, the health indices of the community served by the practice would be comparable with the country as a whole, or with the district in which the practice is located.

Numerator Information.   As indicated, there are several sources of personal health data, but of special relevance in primary health care are the case records of patients and the registration cards of all who are eligible to use the practice. Having decided on the health conditions to be included in special community programs, the routine inclusion of relevant information during interviews and examinations should be allowed for on the regular forms used for patients, or occasionally on special records designed for the purpose. The kinds of charts used in maternal and child centers may readily be modified for epidemiologic purposes while maintaining their functions for individual care. These include records of expectant mothers and the outcome of their pregnancies, and those for child growth and behavior development.

It is seldom that primary health care practice has similar provisions for health examinations of adults in the population they serve. As indicated earlier, the practice may want to develop a community medicine program that focuses on only one health condition, such as hypertension. In this case, special provision for the data relevant to this condition should be made on the record forms of the practice, namely, space for recording repeated systolic and diastolic pressure readings and the clinical complications of hypertension. However, arrangements can also be made for a more comprehensive approach to a community syndrome, such as that in which hypertension, hyperlipidemia, and hyperglycemia are common and are associated with coronary heart disease, cerebral vascular disease, and diabetes mellitus. The record should include provision for these conditions and the personal behavior on which the program is focused, such as cigarette smoking, physical exercise, diet, and medication. In other communities, the associated conditions requiring the attention of community-oriented primary health care may be tuberculosis and malnutrition. In this event, the routines and the records should include special examinations directed toward these disorders.

Whatever data are decided upon, operational definitions of the variables to be recorded should be standardized to ensure as little variation as possible over time and between different recorders. The face sheet of the case record should include information that can be matched with that of the denominator.

Whenever it is proposed to conduct a health survey, it is essential to use sound epidemiologic methods, having available standard texts on the subject, such as that of Abramson.[54]

REFERENCES

1. Morris JN: Community Diagnosis: Community Health. In Uses of Epidemiology, 3rd ed. London, Churchill Livingstone, 1975.
2. McGavran EG: Scientific diagnosis and treatment of the community as a patient. JAMA 162:723, 1956.
3. Kark SL, Kark E: A practice of social medicine. In Kark SL, Steuart GW (eds): A Practice of Social Medicine. Edinburgh, Livingstone, 1962, chap 1.
4. Kark SL: Community health research. Johns Hopkins Med J 124:258, 1969.
5. ———: Epidemiology and Community Medicine. New York, Appleton, 1974.
6. Pearse IH, Williamson GS: The Case for Action. London, Faber & Faber, 1931.
7. Williamson GS, Pearse IH, Staff of the Center: Biologists in Search of Material. London, Faber & Faber, 1938.
8. Pearse IH, Crocker LH: The Peckham Experiment. London, Allen & Unwin, 1943.
9. World Health Organization: The first ten years of the World Health Organization. In The Constitution of the World Health Organization. Geneva, WHO, 1958, p 459.
10. Wan TTH, Livieratos B: Interpreting a general index of subjective well-being. Milbank Mem Fund Q 56:531, 1978.
11. Maddox GL, Douglas EB: Aging and individual differences: a longitudinal analysis of social, psychological and physiological indicators. J Gerontol 29:555, 1974.
12. Court Report: Committee on Child Health Services. Fit for the Future. London, HMSO, 1976.
13. Jenkins GHC, Collins C, and Andrew S: Developmental surveillance in general practice. Br Med J 1:1537, 1978.
14. National Center for Health Statistics: Health Survey Procedure. Vital and Health Statistics. Public Health Service Publication No. 1000, Series 1, No. 2. Washington, D.C., DHEW, 1964.

15. Katz S, Ford AB, Moskowitz RW, et al.: Studies of illness in the aged. The index of ADL. A standardized measure of biological and psychosocial function. JAMA 185:914, 1963.
16. Mahoney FI, Barthel DW: Functional evaluation. The Barthel Index. Md State Med J 14:61, 1965.
17. World Health Organization: International Classification of Diseases, 9th revision. Geneva, WHO, 1977.
18. World Organization of National Colleges, Academics, Academic Associations of General Practitioners/Family Physicians: International Classification of Health Problems in Primary Care (ICH PPC-2). Oxford, Oxford Univ. Press, 1979.
19. Bowlby J: Attachment and Loss. Vol 1. Attachment. London, Hogarth, 1969.
20. Brown GW: Social causes of disease. In Tuckett D (ed): An Introduction to Medical Sociology. London, Tavistock, 1976, chap 9.
21. Medalie JH, Kahn HA, Neufeld HN, et al.: Five-year myocardial infarction incidence. II. Association of single variables to age and birthplace. J Chron Dis 26:329, 1973.
22. Leighton AH: My Name is Legion. New York, Basic, 1959.
23. Parsons T: The Social System. New York, Free Press, 1951.
24. Durkheim E: Suicide. London, Routledge & Kegan Paul, 1952.
25. Cohen AK: Deviance and Control. Englewood Cliffs, New Jersey, Prentice-Hall, 1966.
26. Paul BD (ed): Health, Culture and Community. New York, Russell Sage Foundation, 1955.
27. WHO and UNICEF: The control of acute diarrhoeal diseases: WHO and UNICEF collaborate in country programmes. WHO Chron 33:131, 1979.
28. Shaw CR, McKay HD: Juvenile Delinquency and Urban Areas. Chicago, Univ. of Chicago Press, 1942 (rev. ed. 1969).
29. Park RE, Burgess EW: The City. Chicago, Univ. of Chicago Press, 1925.
30. Burgess EW (ed): The Urban Community. Chicago, Univ. of Chicago Press, 1926.
31. Kaplan BH: A note on religious beliefs and coronary heart disease. J SC Med Assoc Suppl 60, 1976.
32. Comstock GW, Partridge KD: Church attendance and health. J Chron Dis 25:665, 1972.
33. Tumin MM: Social Stratification. Englewood Cliffs, New Jersey, Prentice-Hall, 1967.
34. Eisenstadt SN: Social Differentiation and Stratification. Glenview, Illinois and London, Scott, Foresman, 1971.
35. Edwards AW: Comparative Occupational Statistics for the United States. 16th Census 1940. Washington D.C., GPO, 1943.
36. Office of Population Census and Surveys: Occupational Mortality. The Registrar General's decennial supplement for England and Wales 1970-72. Series DS No. 1. London, HMSO, 1978.
37. Susser MW, Watson W: Sociology in Medicine, 2nd ed. London, Oxford Univ. Press, 1971.
38. Hollingshead AB: The index of social position, In Hollingshead AB, Redlich FC: Social Class and Mental Illness. A Community Study. New York, Wiley, 1958, part 5.

39. Brichler M: Classification of the population by social and economic characteristics. The French experience and international recommendations. J R Stat Soc A 121(2):161, 1958.
40. Reiser SJ: The emergence of the concept of screening for disease. Milbank Mem Fund Q 56:403, 1978.
41. Wilson JMG, Jungner G: Principles and Practice of Screening for Disease. Geneva, WHO, 1968.
42. Nuffield Provincial Hospitals Trust: Screening for Medical Care. London, Oxford Univ. Press, 1968.
43. Cochrane AL: Effectiveness and Efficiency. London, Nuffield Provincial Hospitals Trust, 1972.
44. Holland WW: Taking stock. Lancet 1:1494, 1974.
45. Sackett DL: Screening for early detection of disease: To what purpose? Bull NY Acad Med 51:39, 1975.
46. Shapiro S: Screening for early detection of cancer and heart disease. Bull NY Acad Med 51:80, 1975.
47. Jelliffe DB: The Assessment of the Nutritional Status of the Community. Geneva, WHO Monograph Series 53:1, 1966.
48. Omran AR, Standley CC (eds): Family Formation Patterns and Health. Geneva, WHO, 1976.
49. Hawthorne VM: Epidemiology and treatment of hypertension in the community. Curr Med Res Opin 5:109, 1977.
50. Bryers F, Hawthorne VM: Screening for mild hypertension: costs and benefits. J Epidemiol Community Health 32:171, 1978.
51. Somers AR (ed): The Kaiser-Permanente Medical Care Program: A Symposium. New York, Commonwealth Fund, 1977.
52. Egdahl RH, Friedland J, Mahler AJ, et al.: Fee-for-service health maintenance organizations. JAMA 241:588, 1979.
53. Levitt R: The Reorganised National Health Service, 2nd ed. London, Croom Helm, 1977.
54. Abramson, JH: Survey Methods in Community Medicine, 2nd ed. London–Edinburgh–New York, Churchill Livingstone, 1979.

CHAPTER 3

THE COMMUNITY HEALTH CARE TEAM

The ways in which teamwork have been developed and the composition of the teams have differed according to place and time. They depend on the manpower available, the objectives of the service, and the demands made on it by the community. The important underlying factor is the concept and motivation for the development of community health care.

Physicans and nurses, or alternates for these professional workers, are usually key members of the team. Their usual responsibility is for care of patients, sometimes extending to include care of families, and very seldom to an acceptance of responsibility for care of the community as a whole. Very often, the doctors and nurses providing primary health care for the sick function separately from those who are responsible for primary health care of people who are well. Thus, in many countries, there are separate teams for curative and preventive clinics, both of which may be in the same neighborhood. Social workers, trained as caseworkers, may be additional members of the clinical practice team. The addition of such workers as key members of the primary-care team is an indication of the recognition of the behavioral and social dimension of case management in community health care. Whether social workers should be first-contact practitioners, as are physicians and nurses, or referral personnel is an interesting and important question.

Changing health-related behavior in communities has required extension of the basic team to include community health workers, such as health educators and community organizers. Although their designations differ, their functions have become increasingly recognized.

Their main functions include promoting family and community activities to improve the home and neighborhood.

To establish a joint practice of community medicine and primary health care, the activities of a health care team should focus on individuals and the community with its primary small intimate groups, such as the family, neighborhood, or village, as well as more formal and large secondary groups.[1-3] These activities include personal health care, curative and preventive, and community health work involving community organization, health education, and environmental health services. The extent to which these functions need to be included in a single team varies according to place, state of health of the population, the expressed wishes of the people, and the interests and skills of the health workers. Thus, in a city, the environmental health services may be the function of an engineering and sanitation department, with limited need for environmental health workers as members of the central team of a neighborhood health center. On the other hand, such workers may be of central importance in a rural village health center or in a neglected poverty neighborhood of a city.

Clear definition of the roles of members of a health team is needed to ensure their reciprocal functioning, and the question arises as to whether it is possible to define functions that may have universal relevance. For this purpose, it is helpful to consider the functions for individual care on the one hand and for group and community centered care on the other. Among the main skills required for care of the individual are clinical diagnostic ability, knowledge of appropriate treatment, and its application to the patient. This involves appraisal of the patients' problems, judgment as to the best ways of managing them, and the capacity to establish satisfactory relationships with patients and their families, within the framework of which care of the patient proceeds. Diagnosis and action directed toward the health needs of groups and the community as a whole require different skills, namely, epidemiologic and group-oriented abilities. These two broadly defined aspects of community health care may be developed in different ways in various centers. Most often, the individual clinical aspects are the predominant feature of health care in the community, and the epidemiologic, or group and community health care functions, are separately provided by public health services. More integrated community health care centers, which aim to include important elements of both, need health teams in which both of these broad functions are represented. There are more specific functions within each of these two broadly defined areas. These functions differ in kind and level.

In recent years, much attention has been directed to the primary health care team, especially in its work with individuals and their families. Among the important early reports on the team approach to family medical practice were those of the Montefiore Family Health Maintenance Demonstration in New York City.[4-7] The objectives were to explore the services that could be added to general medical care in order to promote the health of families. Thus, the family practice that was developed combined general curative medical care with preventive and promotive services. The central health team consisted of an internist and pediatrician, a public health nurse, and a psychiatric social worker. The doctors were responsible for patients with physical disease, the public health nurse for the health-relevant aspects of daily family and home life, and the social worker for personal social relationships and adjustment. The functioning of this team will be further reviewed in the discussion on the role of the social worker in primary health care. This central team was supported by two kinds of consultants: medical specialists to whom cases were referred, and advisers to the team in development of the practice, namely, a psychiatrist, social scientist, psychologist, and health educator.

Similarly, a working group of the World Health Organization (European Region) identified the medical practitioner or primary physician, the nurse, and the social worker as the basic members of the primary-care team.[8] The group suggested that this central team might be expanded in several ways. First, the multiple team, in which there may be a group of doctors in primary-care practice with a number of nurses and several social workers. Second, the professionals may include dentists, midwives, pharmacists, and others. Third, the team may include specially trained auxiliaries and assistants, such as medical assistants, auxiliary nurses, midwives, and others.

From the experience of neighborhood health centers established in many disadvantaged poor communities of the United States, Parker[9] perceived the basic nuclear team of these centers as consisting of three professional categories with complementary functions:

1. Primary medical skills of the highest level carried out by primary physicians, who may be general practitioners, internists, or pediatricians.
2. Intermediate level practitioners, that is, professionals who have intermediate levels of responsibility, such as public health nurses, nurse practitioners, or physician's assistants. The responsibility of a worker such as the public health nurse includes supervision of family health workers. It should be noted here that Parker uses the

term "intermediate-level practitioner" differently from the way it is described by us.
3. Family health workers, who are usually residents in the community served by the neighborhood health center. The family health worker goes into the home, carrying out simple treatments and procedures needed in diagnosis, such as blood pressure readings and weighing of babies. She is also the main home health educator, and is, in fact, the bridge from the health center's professional staff to the people in their homes. Being the team member who is closest to the people, she provides the feedback to the team about the family, home, and environment of a patient. Their function in social and environmental intervention is emphasized. There are attributes of this family health worker's role which resemble those to be discussed in more detail later when considering the functions of community health workers, whose major concern is with health-related behavior of the community. They also closely resemble the health visitor described by Adair and Deuschle among the Navajo,[10] and the community health educators of different ethnic groups, trained in South Africa over the period from 1940 to 1959.[3]

THE HEALTH TEAM IN COMMUNITY-ORIENTED PRIMARY HEALTH CARE

The development of a unified practice of community medicine and primary health care needs new health teams. In many Western countries, the usual primary-care services in the community consist of curative services delivered by general practitioners and maternal and child health services conducted by public health nurses. Uniting these two individual or family-centered services into a more comprehensive form of primary care requires a team consisting of three components:

The Central or Nuclear Team.   Physicians, nurses, social caseworkers, and others involved in day-to-day contacts with patients and their families.

Supportive Members of the Team.   Administrators and those whose activities are fundamental to the functioning of the central team, such as health records, laboratory, pharmacy, and secretarial work.

Consultative Members of the Team.   In most cases, such consultative workers will not be members of the team, as the majority of consultations might take place by referral of the patient to another institution. However, consultative functions can, and wherever possible should, be carried out at primary-care centers. In many group practices, as in specialist groups, consultations are conducted by members of the group for one another.

Team Modifications Required for a Community-Oriented Practice.   The team needs to include additional members with special skills in community medicine, such as epidemiology, biostatistics, and health-related behavior, including health education and community organization. It will also need consultants with specialized knowledge of the areas to which the community medicine aspects of the primary-care practice are directed.

The team needed for community-oriented primary health care will thus consist of the following members:

The Central or Nuclear Team

The central team should consist of at least three groups: physicians, nurses, and health educators/community organizers.

The physicians and nurses should be trained in clinical and community health skills. These skills may be effectively combined by some practitioners, such as physicians with both clinical and epidemiologic training, and nurses who are able to care for individual patients, families, and larger groups within the community. On the other hand, these medical and nursing skills can be brought together by complementary functioning of different members of the central team.

The members with skills in health education and community organization require special training to suit them to new functions of a central team in community-oriented primary care. While at least one highly trained worker is required, the function should be conducted by several specially trained community health workers suitable for, or possibly from, the particular community.

Supportive Members of the Team

These will include the same functions as those mentioned for a primary-care center not practicing community medicine. However, the functions of the team members will be modified, especially those of the health recorder, who will be required to provide records not only for case follow-up, but also for epidemiologic purposes, such as community diagnosis, health surveillance, and program evaluation.

Consultative Members of the Team

The consultants will be of two main kinds, those for the care of patients and those for the community medicine aspects of the practice. The latter would ideally include:

Consultants in epidemiology, biostatistics, and health-related behavior.

Consultants in planning and development of specific community programs, such as growth and behavior development of children, mental health, nutrition, or more specifically defined programs concerned with hypertension, heart disease, cancer, obesity, diabetes, tuberculosis, and other communicable diseases.

The Community and the Team

There is a growing movement toward a greater degree of community participation in the conduct of community based health services.

Epidemiologists, biostatisticians, or social scientists concerned with health-related behavior could function in several primary-care teams, thereby extending their skills to a wider population than that of a single primary-care physician or nurse. On the other hand, those who are trained for special functions of community health work, such as health education and community organization, may be needed in greater concentration than primary-care physicians.

There is increasing recognition of the distinctive functions of practitioners who provide primary care in the community. Among the wide variety of such workers, doctors and nurses, their substitutes, social workers, and traditional practitioners will be discussed further, with special reference to their functions in developing a unified practice of community medicine and primary health care. In addition, we will consider the need for special community health workers concerned mainly with health-related behavior of the community.

THE PRIMARY-CARE PRACTITIONER
AS A COMMUNITY PHYSICIAN

When the patients of primary-care physicians constitute a defined population, the practitioners have the opportunity of taking responsibility for the health of the population registered with their practice. As clinicians, they care for those who seek their attention as patients and for those who come for advice, preventive care, or health education. As community physicians, their attention would be centered on particular groups in the community or on the community as a whole. Can each physician carry out these complementary roles of clinician and community physician in a practice, or would it be better to assign the roles to different physicians in a health team? There is no single answer to this question. While the functions are complementary, the skills needed are different: clinical diagnostic ability versus epidemiologic and community diagnostic skills; care and management of a patient versus concern with group and community activities, whether involving care of the sick or promoting the community's health. There are doctors who are willing to undertake both roles. It is not an easy task and requires special motivation, orientation, and training.

Before outlining the proposed functions of physicians in combining the practice of community medicine with their primary care, it is well to consider the role of the community physician in the British National Health Service. The concept of the community physician, like that of community medicine, is relatively new and yet old in its origins.[11] It has its roots in the well-established functions of the medical officer of health (MOH) responsible for the public's health,[12] and emerges from the changes that are taking place, with health care being accepted as a basic right. Hence, public health has extended its functions to the organization of medical care, including primary care in the community and hospital facilities. The role of the community physician is also a response to the emergence of new public health problems: the changing age structure of the population and the consequent increased prevalence of physical and mental chronic diseases with their accompanying disabilities; the increasing recognition of the importance of health surveillance; the care of groups, beyond mothers and children, such as working populations and the aged. With this there has been an extension of the role of public health, in which primary prevention remains fundamental but there are added activities involving the development and organization of health services, available to all according to need rather than ability to pay. Newer and wider concepts of epidemiology have developed and are now needed for community diagnosis and identification of health problems, in the study of medical care, and in evaluation of its effectiveness.[13] The use of controlled clinical trials is being increasingly stressed in order to establish scientific foundations for assessment of various preventive and therapeutic measures before their acceptance and widespread use.[14,15] Community physicians thus need specialized training for their role in the application of epidemiology to decision making in health administration and in their educative and advisory functions.

The roles of the community physician may be national or regional, in urban or rural settings, in large or small communities. The case made by us here is that in the smaller units or local communities, the primary-care practitioner should also be the community physician, thereby combining the practice of community medicine and primary health care.

The Need for Epidemiology
in the Primary Physician's Practice

If primary-care physicians are to extend their practice to include community medicine, they will need some of the additional skills of the community physician. They must be able to investigate and answer the basic questions that face the practitioner of community medicine concerning the state of health of the community, what is being done and what could be done about it, methods of health surveillance, and evaluation of health care. It is very seldom that doctors in primary care give as much attention to answering these questions about the community as they do to similar questions about an individual patient who seeks their care. In order to bring together the clinical and epidemiologic skills needed for practicing community medicine in the framework of their primary health care, practitioners should have training in the principles and methods of epidemiology and its uses in primary health care. This must include experience in a unit in which epidemiology is used in developing such a combined practice.[16-18] To ensure the acceptance of this kind of responsibility, all the primary-care physicians of a health center or group practice should have such training. In addition, one or more of them might have more specialized knowledge in this field, and like the other members who have their additional special skills in various clinical fields, they might function in an advisory and consultant capacity to the group. They would thus guide the practice in regular reviews of progress of the community's health and in the development of special community medicine programs. If at least one of the physicians has more specialized knowledge in epidemiology and community medicine, the group's skills in this wider field of their practice would be improved.

Much of this discussion has been concerned with the primary-care practitioner as a generalist. The reason is the considerable attention recently given to the future of general practice as the basis of primary health care. However, specialists are often involved in providing primary care and episodic crisis care, as well as continuing care of patients. This is especially true in such general specialties as pediatrics, internal medicine, psychiatry, and geriatrics. There is also a body of opinion which holds that with increasing advances in medical knowledge and technology, it has become necessary for all physicians to specialize. One suggestion is that a more satisfactory basis for future primary health care would be the replacement of the general practitioner by a group of personal doctors, namely, obstetrician, pediatrician, internist, and geriatrician. They would conduct their practice in a health center and have responsibility for the preventive and curative aspects of their practices in a defined population, caring for their patients at home, at the health center, or in the hospital, except in those cases where more specialized care was needed.[19] We would add that each needs training in epidemiology and community medicine in order to take responsibility for a community's health.

Group Practice

The day of the solo practitioner is drawing to an end. There is a rapidly growing trend toward practitioners working in groups, from a group practice clinic or a health center. The group may be composed of specialists, or general practitioners, with each member having additional interest and knowledge in a special area of practice. Thus, in addition to conducting their own practices, they are able to provide one another with consultations about cases on which their special experience may be of help, as for a pediatric, geriatric, internal medicine, psychiatric, obstetric, or other problem.[20,21] Each member of the group may have affiliation with a community hospital. Whether a group practice of specialists will be an adequate substitute for the general practitioner or not, it is clear that redefinition of the practitioners' functions will be needed if the group is to combine the practice of community medicine with primary health care. The organization of the medical practice should allow for expanded functions of the practitioners and for the addition of physicians specially qualified in epidemiology and community medicine. A major question that arises here is how general practitioners, or a group practice of specialists, can be assisted to extend their functions to include the second dimension of community health care, namely, the application of epidemiology in a practice aiming to promote the community's health, over and above its functions of personal primary care.

In whatever way the work of physicians is organized, they will not be sufficient in number to staff the future primary health care services, even in the more developed countries. How then can we ask primary-care physicians to extend their clinical practice functions by adding an important role for them in community medicine? By providing them with assistants for clinical work and adding special manpower for community medicine. The community health care team of the kind outlined earlier would answer this question. The development of community medicine in primary care is influenced by, and in fact depends on, the orientation of the physicians in the practice who are key members in the decision-making process in such teams. Without ensuring their training and interest in epidemiology and community medicine, the team will make little progress toward community orientation of primary health care.

THE COMMUNITY NURSE

Working apart from doctors, or together with them, the nurse is well established as a primary health care practitioner. The extent of her independent functioning varies considerably, from a person trained to carry out instructions to one with a considerable degree of autonomy in decision making. In many activities, she is the pivot of community health care, as in the role of public health nurse or health visitor, midwife, or nursing the sick at home. In other situations, she is an assistant to the doctor, giving technical help with medical procedures, such as taking blood samples, giving injections or local treatment, and dressings.

The nurse's roles in community health care extend through care of the individual, the family, and the community, and are carried out in the home, at a clinic or health center, or in institutions in the community, such as schools or community centers. These various roles are often performed by different nurses working in separate agencies.

The Responsibility of the Community Nurse
for Individual Care

Of all community nurses, perhaps the most established independent worker is the midwife. The midwife is a recognized traditional practitioner in many societies, and the association of midwifery training with that of general nursing produces a well-qualified nurse-midwife practitioner. In more developed countries, there is a marked trend toward confinement in hospitals, where many such midwives are employed in addition to obstetricians. However, in extensive areas of the world, domiciliary midwifery and confinement facilities at community health centers are conducted by midwives. They are thus an important professional group of nurses with responsibility for individual care and should be considered an integral part of primary health care teams in the community.

However, independent functioning in care of patients extends to other fields. Nurses have responsibility for primary care of the sick in acute and chronic illness, as well as health appraisal and advice to the well. In many situations, they are the clinical colleagues of physicians, sharing the responsibility of care and perhaps giving more emphasis to the personal aspects. In this way, they help improve the quality of the practice and add to the manpower resources for primary care. In many areas, they work in association with intermediate level medical practitioners, such as the "medical assistant." Often, they are the responsible clinicians in health centers or subcenters, only being in communication with a physician some distance away.

There have been many interesting reports on the role of the nurse in clinical practice, such as rural and family nurse practitioner,[22,23] the pediatric nurse practitioner,[24,25] and similar nurse practitioner programs for adults.[26,27] These have been followed by the establishment of nurse clinics in various parts of the United States, with far-reaching implications for the training of nurses.[28]

The clinical nurse practitioner is not a new concept, but their widespread use in an advanced country like the United States is new. It is therefore important to evaluate the function of a nurse practitioner as a key person in primary-care practice, substituting for or replacing the physician in many situations. Studies have shown that such clinical nurse practitioners are able to conduct an independent general practice and maintain a high level of competence in providing direct patient care.[29-32] A randomized trial in Canada indicates that nurse practitioners are effective and safe for the patients.[33,34] While this development extends clinical resources, there remains a need it apparently does not aim to meet, that of community-oriented primary health care.

The Nurse in a Unified Practice
of Community Medicine and Primary Health Care

In the teamwork of a unified practice of community medicine and primary health care, a more comprehensive family and community nurse practitioner must evolve. As Carolyn Williams aptly states, "There is more to community health nursing than family-oriented care delivered outside the institutional setting; it is a matter of focus on group health problems . . . in contrast to individual, clinically-oriented care."[35]

An approach to expanding the nurse's role in community health care is one that focuses attention on the whole community rather than on the nurse-patient relationship only. The objective is to develop skills in community diagnosis and in action directed toward meeting the community health problems identified. Promoting community health requires skills in group work and appreciation of the community's potential to assume an active role in its own health care.

In many places, the public health nurse has an assignment of a defined area, whether rural village or neighborhood of a city. Among her most important roles is that of ensuring adequate health care of infants, for which purpose she visits the homes of all babies whose births have been registered in that area. This responsibility for the babies of a defined area or community appears to have had its origins with the beginning of the child welfare movement in the United Kingdom in 1862.[36] The Ladies' Health Society of Manchester and Salford was founded at that time by a group of women who were concerned with the unhealthy conditions of the poorer homes in which there were infants. The society employed women to undertake home visiting, with each worker being assigned a district in which she did house-to-house visits. Ways were also sought to obtain information on all births. However, it was more than 25 years later that the system of notification of births to local health authorities was initiated, and still later, in 1907, when the first national Notification of Births Act was passed in that country. The earlier home visitors were replaced by health visitors, who are trained public health nurses. Specialization of functions of the public health nurse developed to meet specific health problems as they were identified, such as school health services and tuberculosis control. In working toward a more comprehensive role for community nursing in primary health care, the well-founded community orientation of public health nursing is a useful starting point.

There is need for community and family nursing as an integral part of community-oriented primary health care. It should combine the functions of public health nurses, with their promotive and preventive roles, the nurse practitioner and clinic nurse, and those of the visiting or district nurse concerned with domiciliary care of the sick. This can be done by a single generalist nurse combining these functions, or by a group of nurses having complementary functions. The concept of community health nursing is evolving to meet the wider functions needed for community health care.[35,37-39] In various health teams with which the writer has been associated in communities of different ethnic groups in South Africa, two such nurses were allocated a defined neighborhood of families, for which they had comprehensive nursing responsibility. The two nurses were linked with one family physician as members of the central team, together with specially trained community health workers.[3,37]

In our work toward a unified practice of primary health care and community medicine in Jerusalem, promotive, preventive, and curative nursing functions have been combined at the health center and in domiciliary care. This has involved further training and considerable modification of traditional roles of public health nursing in this country. Among the important developments are:

Each nurse has responsibilities for a defined area of homes. These include:

1. Conducting independent consultations and examinations of infants and young children at special sessions at the health center, as well as interviews with patients seeking her advice.
2. Conducting systematic follow-up clinics for all the adults of her families who are included in the community medicine program concerned with primary and secondary prevention of cardiovascular disease.
3. Carrying out treatment prescribed by a doctor and other nursing routines, including explanation of treatments, dietary and other advice, taking blood and other specimens for examination, giving injections, dressing wounds, giving gynecologic treatments, and taking anthropometric and blood pressure measurements.
4. Home visits to mothers who have recently returned from hospital and examination of their newly born babies.
5. Follow-up of cases with communicable disease to ensure that proper care is being given, and to prevent spread of the infection.
6. Home care of the chronically sick with special reference to needs of homebound patients, for whom she might call in the assistance of others such as a physiotherapist, occupational therapist, or social worker.
7. She also visits patients of her families while in hospital, and follows up at home afterward if necessary.
8. She conducts health surveys and nursing surveillance, including a periodic home health census of homes in her area. In this way, the health center aims to ensure contact with all homes in the practice and not only those under active treatment. Effective use of such home visits leads to detection of new cases needing care: identification of health-related behavior that may need change or planning a program with the family to effect necessary changes; assessment of the environs and material resources of the home; understanding of family relationships and implications for care, such as child rearing, wife beating, or coping with an aged person in need of long-term care at home.
9. In addition, some of the nurses have responsibilities in the neighborhood schools. Among these are periodic measurements of height and weight, screening procedures including audiometry and tests

of vision, assisting physicians at initial school health examinations, immunization, health education including sex education, and visits to the homes of children when required. The nurse also participates in psychiatric conferences about children with learning and behavior problems. This is done by a special team consisting of the teacher, nurse, social worker, school psychologist, physician, and child psychiatrist.

ALTERNATES FOR PHYSICIANS AND NURSES IN COMMUNITY HEALTH CARE

There are not enough doctors or trained nurses to provide for community health care. The need for alternative arrangements is leading to universal acceptance of the idea of using less-trained manpower. Its recognition by the World Health Organization should go far toward clarifying the kinds of skills and the training required.[40-44]

Intermediate Level Practitioners

The medical assistant and the practical nurse have been used as alternates for doctors and nurses in order to make personal health care more widely available. The use of such workers in community health care has existed for a long time in some parts of the world, but it is only relatively recently that the urgency of the need on a worldwide scale has been recognized. Hence the increasing interest in the potential of such workers, both as replacements and as assistants to doctors and nurses. They have a place in primary health care teams working alongside the more qualified professional, but they also have a place as independent workers in clinics and health centers in the vast areas of the world in which there are no highly qualified practitioners to undertake basic clinical functions of community health care.

The clinical functions of doctor or nurse alternates are considered together because they are often not readily distinguishable. Thus, in one country, work carried out by a practical nurse is much the same as that carried out by a medical assistant in another. For example, the role of practical nurses stationed in rural settlements in Israel has developed in some centers to include clinical functions of a first-contact practitioner. They deal with some cases themselves, refer others to the doctor at the health center, and follow up the doctor's instructions in patient care, either at the patient's home or at their clinic.[45-47] Their primary-care functions are similar to those of medical assistants described in other countries. Thus, the practical nurse who substitutes for the more highly qualified state-registered nurse or public health nurse of Israel is also functioning as a physician's assistant.

There are various levels of responsibility delegated to such workers, and hence there are wide disparities in their training. In addition to the pediatric nurse practitioner discussed earlier, a new type of pediatric practitioner, the child health associate, is being trained in the United States at the University of Colorado Medical Center.[48-50] The training is at university level, requiring 2 years in an undergraduate college, a further 2 years at the university's medical center and a 1 year internship. Child health associates take considerable responsibilities in primary health care, in the care of well children, and in treatment of the sick child, working together with pediatricians, general practitioners, or public health physicians. As described, the child health associate would, in fact, appear to be a practitioner with a lower level of education in pediatric practice than the specialized pediatrician of the United States, but probably with a higher standard of pediatrics than that of the general practitioner in many countries.

Among the oldest and best known of the more highly qualified intermediate level practitioners are the feldshers and feldsher-midwives of the U.S.S.R. They attend special middle-grade medical schools for several years, depending on their standard of schooling, and are expected to provide adequate medical care to patients in the absence of a physician.[51] In more recent years, middle-level practitioners with clinical functions and special training for the purpose have been trained in the United States, with special emphasis on the needs of primary ambulatory medical care. We have already reviewed two of these, the clinical nurse practitioner and the child health associate. The training of physicians' assistants and other new health practitioners has also been developed.[52-55] Their role involves the ability to take a medical history, carry out a physical examination and common laboratory tests, maintain adequate records of case management, and provide care and treatment for defined conditions, including preventive measures. Ability to identify and refer patients needing more skilled evaluation and treatment, to assist the physician in carrying out treatments, and to maintain the progress of patients under care are central features of their function.

Practical nurses function independently in certain situations, but are also extensively employed in both hospital and community health services, working under the direction of more highly trained nurses. Similarly, there is much scope for the employment of intermediate-level medical practitioners in community health centers or clinics, carrying out clinical and community medicine functions as members of a health team together with physicians.

If such intermediate-level workers are to extend their functions beyond individual patient care to concern with the community as a whole, or subgroups within it, they need training in the elements of community health. This would include the principles of epidemiology and its application to primary health care, elementary statistics, and relevant aspects of the social sciences. A period of clerkship in a health center, which is both a practicing and teaching unit in community health care, is essential.

Village Health Worker.   A different kind of need is presented by communities in isolated areas where there is no physician, nurse, or intermediate-level practitioner providing primary care. The introduction of village health workers has been a response to this situation.[56-58] Their functions often go beyond simple medical treatment of common diseases and first aid to other activities involving health education, preventive immunizations, and sometimes specific sanitary measures. In many programs, these village health workers, elected by the village, have a short introductory training before commencing their work, followed by subsequent courses of training. Special elementary texts have been written for use in their training and as guides in their work.[59,60]

The combination of clinical and community orientation by such village health workers is of interest, and this will be discussed further in our consideration of the role of community health workers.

THE SOCIAL WORKER

Like the nurse and doctor, the social worker may function at the individual, family, and community level. The functions of professional trained social workers in the community are usually carried out in the framework of social services, organized and directed separately from the health service organization. This extends through the greatest part of personal social services concerned with individual and family care, as well as community organization and community development. However, social work and health care are in many ways complementary services in society, and it is not surprising that social workers are often concerned with clients who are, at the same time, patients of doctors and nurses. Hence, there is a need to coordinate and, if possible, to integrate the functions of social and health services in the community. This would be of great help to families and individuals, while providing a more holistic and satisfying setting for the workers themselves.

Important elements of social work are practiced in the framework of health services, such as the widely accepted role of the medical social worker in hospitals and the psychiatric social worker in both adult and child psychiatry units in hospitals and in the community. Of special interest here is the potential role of social workers in community health care. Primary health care in the community is increasingly concerned with care of the chronically sick, including care of ambulatory patients and home care of housebound patients. Long-term illness, often associated with aging, involves disabilities, with associated stress and behavior problems in both the disabled individual and the family. The disabled person needs supportive treatment, and the family members, involved as they are in the patient's care, need material help, guidance and education in management, and support in handling their relationships with the patient and with one another. While both the doctor and nurse in primary health care should be trained in the psychologic and social aspects of patient and family care, the specially trained social worker has a most important contribution to make. This might be in direct contact with patients and families, as well as indirectly through advice and interaction with doctors and nurses of the team.

Ensuring the successful integration of the social worker into a primary health care team demands careful attention to several factors. Among these are the community's perception of the role of a worker who is not usually associated with primary health care. Another aspect needing attention is the functional relationship between the social worker, public health nurse, and doctor. Special training programs will be needed for social workers to function in primary health care teams.

An early exploration in integrating a social worker as a member of a primary health care team was that of the Family Health Maintenance Demonstration, conducted by the Montefiore Hospital in New York City.[7,61] Working together with doctor and nurse, the social worker was to be a family caseworker and team member. Thus, she conducted interviews of family members as part of the initial examination of those who were accepted into the program. The expectation of the project was that she would be as much a primary-care team member as were the doctor and nurse, and in addition to her interviews with family members, both she and the public health nurse would visit homes and school.

Generally, social work was not seen by patients as being a part of health services, despite explanations of its functions and the status accorded to the worker at conferences of the health team with the family. There was resistance to acceptance of the need for use of the social worker's service, especially by the less educated and lower occupational groups. The role, being associated with a stereotype of a worker concerned with welfare, mental illness, or disturbed family situations, was not readily acceptable in a primary-care setting usually associated with physical health. The patients' perceptions of the role and utilization of the social worker and others in the team was reported by the social scientist of the project.[62-64] He contrasted the general acceptance of the nurse with that of the social worker. The public health nurse was seen to be a health worker responsible to the doctor and concerned with problems of everyday living with which the housewives were familiar, such as sleeping arrangements, crowding, feeding, and various aspects of homemaking. "In all, the nurse was considered the only person who knew what things were really like at home."[7] Thus, when they had family or emotional problems to discuss, it was natural to discuss them with her. The social worker, on the other hand, was seen as a professional with specialized functions, removed from medical problems, and not familiar with home or school problems, as she rarely visited them. This perception was manifested in a number of ways. For example, at a team case conference with patients, even in matters in which the social worker was best equipped to discuss particular questions, "the patient ignored her and addressed his questions to the physician."[7] Clearly, patients have an important function in determining the role of professional health workers, especially when the worker is new to the situation.

Attachment of social workers to primary health care units has continued to be explored in respect of the contribution such a worker can make in casework with families and individual patients, and as a link between the primary-care team and other community resources.[65] The role of such a worker in dealing with patients' social and psychologic problems has been evaluated by a comparative study of several general practices in London.[66] A social worker was attached to the study or experimental practice, the others functioning as control practices. The results of the trial were encouraging in that over a period of 1 year, the scores of social adjustment and clinical psychiatric state of patients in the experimental practice improved more than did those of similar patients in the control general practices. The positive findings of this evaluative study in a general medical practice not only support the argument for inclusion of social workers in primary health care teams in such communities, but also lead to consideration of the potential of primary health care in community psychiatry.[67]

This review of the social worker's role in primary health care has been restricted to the casework functions with individual patients and their families. The role of the social worker in community organization is considered further in the discussion on the community health worker.

THE COMMUNITY HEALTH WORKER

A joint practice of community medicine and primary health care includes personal health care and community health work involving community organization, health education, and environmental health. The emphasis of the practice will vary according to place, state of health of the community, what the community itself wants, and the skills of the health workers.

As key personal health "carers" in community-oriented primary health care, doctors and nurses need to understand health-related behavior, since an important part of their work is directed toward changing behavior when necessary. Nevertheless, there is little doubt that the behavioral aspects of community health care need the attention of a special worker. We have already reviewed the contribution social caseworkers can make to meet this need in care of patients and their families. The question with which we are now concerned is that of promoting behavior that will ensure the highest possible standard of community health. Community health workers trained to carry out this function should be members of primary health care teams. Their role in health surveillance, in health education, and in involving the community in action promotive of its health should be a vital part of present-day community health care.

The varied functions of community health workers have been in response to different health needs as perceived by health authorities or enterprising individual doctors and nurses. This explains the diversity of roles carried out by community health workers in various countries.

Many years ago, community health workers were trained to carry out specific tasks in well-defined public health programs, directed toward the control of such diseases as malaria and smallpox. Such workers continue in these programs, covering large populations living in widespread regions. The programs are usually conducted under the highly centralized control of experts in the particular disease. For example, in malaria control, the tasks of the field health workers have included home visits, examination of family members for fever and taking of blood specimens, inspection of houses and their environs for the presence of mosquitoes and their breeding places, distribution of prophylactic medicines, simple treatments, health education, and active measures against the mosquito vectors. Surveillance and educational programs carried out by workers trained for a specific purpose are a feature of public health control measures and are being extended into various areas of activity, as in the control and treatment of trachoma.[68]

On the basis of the successful experience gained in such public health projects, it was proposed that a similarly selective, but multipurpose, program of demographic and epidemiologic surveillance be established. The system of domiciliary visits by specially trained workers, as part of the control of a single disease, might thus be extended by adding other specific tasks for such field workers.[69]

While the above developments are of much importance, the main focus of attention in this presentation is on the potential role of community health workers as members of a health team concerned with a unified practice of individual and community health care. Realization of the importance of organizing more comprehensive health care in the community goes back many years,[70,71] and is associated with the use of specially trained community health workers.[3,10,40,41]

Community health workers are often appointed from among the people served by the health care service. There is a strong movement for communities to elect persons from their own communities as community health workers. These workers then undergo various periods of training. They may be voluntary or paid, part-time or full-time, and the size of the population with whom they work varies considerably. They are accountable to the community and may be seen as the spearhead of community participation in its health care.[57,72-77] While this development is being vigorously promoted in developing countries, it was an outstanding feature of the neighborhood health centers established by the Office of Economic Opportunity (OEO) in the United States in the 1960s. Local community family health workers were trained and used by the pioneer OEO neighborhood health centers.[9,78]

The Community Health Worker's Role in Community-Oriented Primary Health Care

Should community health workers fulfill distinctive roles in the practice, or should their role be that of clinical assistants to doctors or nurses? The viewpoint expressed here is that they have a distinctive contribution to make, without which the community medicine aspects of health care will not be effectively developed. Wherever the need for these workers has been recognized, the agency has defined their role and has developed its own program to train them. The training ranges from instruction in carrying out simple tasks to much more sophisticated programs. Doctors and nurses are often responsible for both the training and direction of such workers. Consequently, the more knowledge these doctors and nurses have of epidemiology and community medicine, and the more influenced they are by modern concepts of health education and applied behavioral sciences, the better they will train the community health worker in motivating communities to undertake activities promotive of their health. Thus, it is important that community health care teams as a whole should be exposed to the work of epidemiologists and behavioral scientists who have a special interest in the application of their various fields to community health care.[10,16,79,80]

While community health workers might address themselves to some aspects of individual care, the main thrust of their work should be oriented toward the community as a whole or its important subgroups. Suggestions for the scope of work and central functions of these workers will be considered in relation to the cardinal questions that face the health team practicing community medicine.

Collecting Data for Community Diagnosis.   In answering the questions, What is the state of health of the community? and What are the factors responsible for this state of health? the role of the community health worker includes such activities as:

> Gathering data on the population, which will allow for analysis of associations between various demographic attributes and health characteristics. Thus, by household surveys, it is possible to obtain demographic data such as age and sex, family composition and family spacing, perceived health status of individual family members.
>
> Surveys of health-related behavior. The behavior investigated will depend on the health problems that have been identified. Common areas of importance are child-rearing practices, dietary practices of different groups, sanitary habits and control of the environment, physical exercise, and smoking. No less important than these investigations of overt behavior are studies of knowledge and attitudes about health and disease, including family planning.

Systematic and continuing study of the community's concepts of its main health problems and of the main factors thought to be promotive of health.

Similarly, the community health worker will help the team answer the questions: What is being done about the health of the community by the community itself and by the health services? This requires:

Gathering information on the functioning of various kinds of health services and the various practitioners, including traditional practitioners.

Finding out about use of health services, especially by different age and sex groups and by other characteristics of the community.

Learning about the perception and expectations the community has of the health services and the emphasis placed on the needs of different groups.

Ascertaining how members of the community perceive their participation in the promotion of their own health care.

With this knowledge, and that gained by other members of the team, decisions can be made as to the action to be taken and its expected outcome. Community health care consists of three component elements: action that has a direct impact on the health of the community, such as immunization and medical treatment; action having an impact on health by modifying the community's health-related behavior, such as changing infant feeding practices; and action directed toward improving the environment in order to prevent disease.

The content of the community health worker's activities would depend on the program decided upon by the health team as a whole. Specific objectives are vital to the success of such work. The main skills needed by the community health worker for this are community health education and promotion of community organization. It also involves liaison work between the community and the health services.

Health Education.   Study of health-relevant behavior and encouraging behavior promotive of health are the central health education tasks of community health workers.

Community Organization or Community Development.   Using community organizations or informal groupings, the community health worker's role is in promoting community participation in identifying and solving its health problems.

Liaison and Interpretation.   As a member of the health team and of the community, the community health worker can readily have a most important liaison and interpretive function between the community and the health service itself, as well as with economic, welfare, education, and other agencies.[10]

"Clinical" and Individual Care.   There are situations where community health workers trained to carry out elementary diagnosis and treatment are most important. A basic question is the extent to which such clinical functions should be developed as part of the community health workers' role. A major problem is that clinical work is often given priority and carried on at the expense of community health work.

Among the important questions that face the health team practicing community medicine are the measures needed for continuing surveillance of the community's health and of the health care being provided, together with evaluation of the action carried out. Here we will discuss the role of the community health worker in these functions.

Surveillance of Health.   Surveillance is the ongoing monitoring of the health status of the population. By periodic surveys or continuing observation and updating of information, the community health worker is able to monitor much of the community's health status and important changes in it. This requires continuing contact with families in the community for recording changes in demography, health-relevant behavior, and the environment.

Evaluation of Programs.   Evaluation of a program requires a clear statement of the purpose and general objectives of that program, together with details of specific measurable objectives, in order to be able to ascertain whether these objectives have been achieved. It involves appraisal of the extent to which the health team is carrying out the program; assessing the response of the community by measurement of changes in its behavior and involvement of its members in the program; measuring the effectiveness of the program in terms of outcome, as shown by changes in the community's state of health; and assessment of its efficiency, especially its efficient use of manpower resources and its cost.

The information obtained by the community health worker for this purpose must be directly relevant to the objectives of the program. Thus, if the objectives include changes in health-relevant behavior, the particular desired behavior needs to be reviewed by periodic surveys or ongoing observation.

THE TRADITIONAL PRACTITIONER

Many years ago, at the celebration of the anniversary of our health center in a rural African community, one of the speakers was an influential tribal chief in whose area the health center was situated, and where the health team lived. He spoke with much warmth of the work of the doctors, nurses, and community health workers, paying equal tribute to our medical, social, and educational interests and activities. He, nevertheless, found something missing in the structure and functioning of the health team. Why was there no place for traditional practitioners, herbalists, and witch doctors in our team? The traditional practitioners knew so much of the ways of thinking, feelings, and actions of the sick and their families; they understood the social situations in which disease was caused, and could, therefore, be prevented and treated. He made a proposal that we should celebrate this anniversary by appointing at least one of the traditional practitioners as an important member of our team. Except for the fact that the law of the land forbade a registered medical practitioner to practice with such unqualified practitioners, it would have been a most interesting experience to have one or more of them on the health team. A number were themselves our patients, they often referred their patients to us, and many patients and families in our health center program were also under their care. Case studies of the health center team had shown their importance in the medical care system of the community.[3,81]

What particular attributes of the local traditional practitioners would have made a positive contribution to the health team's functioning, and in what ways might we have modified their practice to the advantage of the community? The traditional practitioners of the area were an integral part of the communities living there. Their practice was consistent with the community's belief system about the nature and causes of disease, its prevention, and ways of treatment. On the other hand, the clinical team of the health center—doctors, medical aides, and nurses—were trained in modern scientific-based schools and hospitals. Although the majority were themselves Africans whose home language was the same as that of the community's, more important was the fact that their training and practice were essentially Western, and not in accord with the health and disease concepts and customary practices of the local people. This remained essentially true of our team, even when it was extended to include a number of community health workers, who were members of the community itself. While they constituted an important bridge between the health center and the community, their orientation and functions as agents of change in health-related behavior distinguished them, and the team as a whole, from the traditional practitioners, who were a conservative force. Steeped in the local culture, especially in its medical system, the conservativism of the traditional practitioners was itself a major contribution to the health team's practice in care of the individual patient and in its community work. Understanding their orientation and management of disease was to gain insight into the community's concepts and practices, and with this growth in the health team's knowledge, our approach to patients, families, and the community was modified. This extended through to changes in patient-practitioner relationships, the nature of consultations, and ways of reaching a diagnosis. In identifying the main health problems of families and of the community, and the actions we proposed, it was essential to link our framework of thinking about health and disease with that of the community and its traditional practitioners.

There are areas of real disagreement between modern and traditional practice, and at times points of serious conflict in interpretation and the kind of intervention. Ignoring the existence of the traditional practitioner, who is the mooring point during periods of stress or illness of people, is no contribution to the resolution of such conflict. The patient possessed by evil spirits sent by an ill-wisher is not helped by denial of "possession." The family whose illnesses are caused by the spirits of the ancestors, as punishment for transgressions against expected behavior, is not helped by rejection of such expression of social and psychologic illness. Such people look for treatment from the traditional practitioner. As a member of a health team, he might transmit this body of knowledge to the modern practitioners of the team, at the same time being influenced by them. This might reduce the distance between the health team and the community, helping to promote more effective communication in cross-cultural situations.

While the skills and knowledge of traditional practitioners are specific to the communities in which they practice, it is equally true to say that traditional medicine has universal attributes. Traditional practitioners are probably the main providers of primary medical care to the majority of people in the world. Their potential importance for the future health care systems in various parts of the world is being increasingly recognized. There are many difficulties in trying to bridge the differences between scientific and traditional medicine, but this does not mean that it is not desirable or possible to do so. In a discussion on traditional African cultures and Western medicine, Lambo has emphasized the importance of finding compromises that will allow for the integration of some elements of traditional medicine with Western medicine in Africa. He has reported on his experience in collaborating with traditional practitioners in his innovative psychiatric day hospital at Aro, Nigeria.[82,83]

A feature common to African and other peoples' traditional concepts of health and disease is the important role assigned to social phenomena. Living in harmony with one's neighbors and according to the laws of the society and its supernatural world, is the key to protection of one's family and self from disease. Although the conceptual framework of Western medicine is predominantly biologic, there has been considerable development in social medicine and its related disciplines toward understanding the social and cultural processes in the epidemiology of health and disease, and in health care. Thus, there would seem to be both a philosophic and scientific framework in which to proceed with bridging the differences between the biologic orientations of modern medicine and the more social and cultural concepts of traditional medicine.

Yet another aspect of much relevance is the acceptance of supernatural as well as natural theories on the causation of disease.[84] The link between the social and the supernatural, as in the practice of witchcraft, has been the subject of many studies. In Evans-Pritchard's classic study, *Witchcraft, Oracles and Magic Among the Azande,* he not only detailed the stuff of which witchcraft substance is made and the practices of witch doctors, but also the social functions of witchcraft. Not only do beliefs in witchcraft control conduct, but the circumstances in which it is used are succinctly summarized in his expression, "men bewitch others when they hate them."[85] We believe such studies compel the attention of those who seek to develop a practice of community medicine together with primary health care. At the very least, there is need for understanding the knowledge, attitudes, and practices of traditional practitioners within the particular communities in which health care units are being developed. Beyond that, there is the probable usefulness of collaboration with traditional practitioners.

This discussion on the potential role of the traditional practitioner in community health care has been related mainly to traditional African medicine. We have done this because of personal experience in several African communities. The same comments, possibly even more valid, could no doubt be made in respect of such highly organized traditional systems of medicine as Ayuvedic medicine of India and Chinese medicine. The inclusion of the essentials of Ayuvedic medicine in a modern medical curriculum has been discussed, as has the possibility of integrating the large numbers of practitioners of Ayuvedic medicine into the health care system of the country.[86] From China, there are reports on the increasing integration of doctors of traditional Chinese medicine into the health services framework and on its inclusion in the training of future doctors.[87-90]

The fact is that in extensive areas of the world, the greatest part of primary care is provided by traditional practitioners of folk medicine. While the nature of their practice varies from place to place, they constitute a universal system of medical care. Those who plan to introduce modern health care in the community need to be aware of the universality of the traditional practitioner. There is no community that does not have its "traditional" health care system, and it is the task of the innovator to identify it and consider its incorporation, so as to ensure community involvement and participation in building toward a more comprehensive development of community health care.

REFERENCES

1. Cooley CH: Social Organization. New York, Schocken, 1962 (first published 1909, Scribner's).
2. Davis K: Human Society. New York, Macmillan, 1973.
3. Kark SL, Steuart GW (eds): A Practice of Social Medicine. Edinburgh, Livingstone, 1962.
4. Cherkasky M: The Family Health Maintenance Demonstration, in Research in Public Health. New York, Milbank Memorial Fund, 1952.
5. Milbank Memorial Fund: The Family Health Maintenance Demonstration. Report of a Round Table Conference. New York, Milbank Memorial Fund, 1954.
6. Silver GA: Beyond general practice: the health team. Yale J Biol Med 31:29, 1958.
7. ———: Family Medical Care. A Report on the Family Health Maintenance Demonstration. Cambridge, Harvard Univ. Press, 1963.
8. World Health Organization: Trends in the Development of Primary Care. Report on a Working Group Convened by the Regional Office for Europe of the WHO. Regional Office for Europe. Copenhagen, WHO, 1973.
9. Parker AW: The Team Approach to Primary Health Care. Berkeley, Univ. of California, 1972.
10. Adair J, Deuschle KW: The People's Health. Medicine and Anthropology in a Navajo Community. New York, Appleton, 1970.
11. Charles J: On the State of the Public Health for the Year 1959. London, Ministry of Health, HMSO, 1960.
12. Morris JN: Tomorrow's community physician. Lancet 2:811, 1969.
13. ———: Uses of Epidemiology, 3rd ed. Edinburgh, London, Livingstone, 1975.
14. Cochrane AL: Effectiveness and Efficiency. Nuffield Provincial Hospitals Trust, 1972.

15. Abramson JH. The four basic types of evaluation: clinical reviews, clinical trials, program reviews, and program trials. Public Health Rep 94:210, 1979.
16. Kark SL: Community Medicine and Primary Health Care. In Epidemiology and Community Medicine. New York, Appleton, 1974, Sec 5.
17. Hart JT: The marriage of primary care and epidemiology. J R Coll Physicians 8:299, 1974.
18. Kark SL, Kark E, Hopp C, et al.: The control of hypertension, atherosclerotic disease and diabetes in a family practice. J R Coll Gen Pract 26:157, 1976.
19. McKeown T: Medicine in Modern Society. London, Allen & Unwin, 1965.
20. Silver GA: A Spy in the House of Medicine. Germantown, Maryland, Aspen Systems, 1976.
21. Bain DJG: Health Centre Practice in Livingstone, New Town. Health Bull (Edinb) 31:290, 1973.
22. Sullivan JA, Dachelet CZ, Sultz HA, et al.: The rural nurse practitioner: a challenge and a response. Am J Public Health 68:972, 1978.
23. Pesznecher BL, Draye MA: Family nurse practitioners in primary care: a study of practice and patients. Am J Public Health 68:977, 1978.
24. Silver HK, Ford LC, Stearly SG: A program to increase health care for children: the pediatric nurse practitioner program. Pediatrics 39:756, 1967.
25. ——, Ford LC, Day LR: The pediatric nurse practitioner program: expanding the role of the nurse to provide increased health care for children. JAMA 204:298, 1968.
26. Lewis, CE, Resnik BA: Nurse clinics and ambulatory patient care. N Engl J Med 277:1236, 1967.
27. ——, Resnik BA, Schmidt G, et al.: Activities, events and outcomes in ambulatory patient care. N Engl J Med 280:645, 1969.
28. Secretary's Committee Report: Extending the Scope of Nursing Practice. A Report by a Special Committee to the Secretary, Department of Health, Education and Welfare. Am J Nurs 71:2346, 1971.
29. Duncan B, Smith AN, Silver HK: Comparison of the physical assessment of children by pediatric nurse practitioners and pediatricians. Am J Public Health 61:1170, 1971.
30. Charney E, Kitzman H: The child health nurse (pediatric nurse practitioner) in private practice. A controlled trial. N Engl J Med 285:1353, 1971.
31. Chappell JA, Drogos PA: Evaluation of infant health care by a nurse practitioner. Pediatrics 49:871, 1972.
32. Taller SL, Feldman R: The training and utilization of nurse practitioners in adult health appraisal. Med Care 12:40, 1974.
33. Spitzer WO, Sackett DL, Sibley JC, et al.: The Burlington randomized trial of the nurse practitioner. N Engl J Med 290:251, 1974.
34. Sackett DL, Spitzer WO, Gent M, et al.: The Burlington randomized trial of the nurse practitioner: Health outcomes of patients. Ann Intern Med 80:137, 1974.
35. Williams C: Community health nursing—what is it? Nurs Outlook 25:250, 1977.
36. Lane-Claypon JE: The Child Welfare Movement. London, Bell, 1920.
37. Cohn HD: Family and Community Nursing. In Kark SL, Steuart GW (eds): A Practice of Social Medicine. Edinburgh, Livingstone, 1962, chap 2.

38. WHO Expert Committee Report: Community Health Nursing. Geneva, WHO, 1974.
39. Skrovan C, Anderson ET, Gottschalk J: Community nurse practitioner: an emerging role. Am J Public Health 64:847, 1974.
40. Fendall NRE: The Auxiliary in Medicine. In Prywes M, Davies M (eds): Health Problems in Developing States. New York, Grune & Stratton, 1968, p 294.
41. ———: Auxiliaries in Health Care: Programs in Developing Countries. Baltimore, Josiah Macy Foundation, Johns Hopkins Press, 1972.
42. Rosinski EF, Spencer FJ: The training and duties of the medical auxiliary known as the assistant medical officer. Am J Public Health 57:1663, 1967.
43. Pitcairn, DM, Flahault D (eds): The Medical Assistant: An Intermediate Level of Health Care Personnel. Geneva, WHO, 1974.
44. Watson EJ: Meeting community health needs: the role of the medical assistant. WHO Chron 30:91, 1976.
45. Arnon A: Comprehensive family medicine in a rural area. Aust Fam Physician 2:256, 1973.
46. ———: Family medicine at the Nehora Health Centre (in Hebrew with English and French summaries). Fam Physician 1:80, 1971.
47. Yodfat Y: A new method of teamwork in family medicine in Israel with the participation of nurses as physician's assistants. Am J Public Health 62:953, 1972.
48. Silver HK, Ott JE: The child health associate: a new health professional to provide comprehensive health care to children. Pediatrics 51:1, 1973.
49. Fine LL, Scriven SS: The child health associate: a non-physician primary care practitioner for children. The P A Journal 7:137, 1977.
50. AMA Department of Health Manpower: The child health associate: a new training program in Colorado. JAMA 212:1045, 1970.
51. Ministry of Health of the U.S.S.R.: The Training and Utilization of Feldshers in the U.S.S.R. Public Health Papers No. 56. Geneva, WHO, 1974.
52. Lippard V, Purcell E (eds): Intermediate Level Health Practitioners. New York, Josiah Macy Foundation, 1973.
53. Sadler AM: The new health practitioner in primary care. J Med Educ 49:845, 1974.
54. ——— AM: New health practitioner education: problems and issues. J Med Educ 50:67 (part 2), 1975.
55. Hudson JI, Nourse ES (eds): Perspectives in primary care education. J Med Educ 50 (part 2), 1975.
56. Harrison TJ: Training village health aides in the Kodzebul area of Alaska. Public Health Rep 80:565, 1965.
57. Djukanovic V, Mach EP (eds): Alternative Approaches to Meeting Basic Health Needs in Developing Countries. Geneva, WHO, 1975.
58. Smith AJ: Medicine in China. Barefoot doctors and the medical pyramid. Br Med J 2:429, 1974.
59. Werner D: Where There Is No Doctor, a Village Health Care Handbook. Palo Alto, California, The Hesperian Foundation, 1977.
60. World Health Organization: The Primary Health Worker. Geneva, WHO, 1977.
61. Silver GA: Family Medical Care: A Design for Health Maintenance. Cambridge, Massachusetts, Ballinger, 1974.

62. Freidson E: Social science research in the family health maintenance demonstration. In Silver GA: Family Medical Care. Cambridge, Harvard Univ. Press, 1963, p 227.

63. Freidson E: Patients' Views of Medical Practice. New York, Russell Sage Foundation, 1961.

64. ———: Specialties without roots: the utilization of new services. Human Organization 18:112, 1959.

65. Goldberg EM, Neill JE: Social Work in General Practice. London, Allen & Unwin, 1973.

66. Cooper B, Harwin BG, Depla C, et al.: Mental health care in the community: an evaluative study. Psychol Med 5:371, 1975.

67. World Health Organization: Psychiatry and Primary Medical Care. Copenhagen, WHO Regional Office for Europe, 1973.

68. Willard N: Eye team in action. World Health, February–March 1976.

69. Frederiksen HS: Epidemographic Surveillance. Monograph 13. Chapel Hill, Carolina Population Center, Univ. of North Carolina, 1971.

70. Lord Dawson of Penn: The Dawson Interim Report on the Future Provision of Medical and Allied Health Services. London, HMSO, 1920 (reprinted 1950).

71. Seipp C (ed): Health Care for the Community. Selected Papers of Dr. John B. Grant. Baltimore, Johns Hopkins Press, 1963.

72. Hughes JP (ed): Health Care for Remote Areas. Oakland, Kaiser Foundation, 1972.

73. Newell K (ed): Health by the People. Geneva, WHO, 1975.

74. McNeur RW (ed): The Changing Roles and Education of Health Care Personnel Worldwide in View of the Increase of Basic Health Services. Philadelphia, Society for Health and Human Values, 1978.

75. World Health Organization: India: a new class of community health workers. World Health, April 1978, p 30.

76. Tarimo E: Health and self-reliance: the experience of Tanzania. Development Dialogue 1:35, 1978.

77. Chowdhury Z: The paramedics of Savar: an experiment in community health in Bangladesh. Development Dialogue 1:41, 1978.

78. Office of Health Affairs: Team Approach to Health Care in Neighborhood Health Centers. Proceedings of the Third Training Conference. Washington, D.C., Office of Health Affairs, OEO, December 1968.

79. Foster GM: Applied Anthropology. Boston, Little, Brown, 1969.

80. Steuart GW: Community health education. In Kark SL, Steuart GW (eds): A Practice of Social Medicine. Edinburgh, Livingstone, 1962, chap 3.

81. Cassell J: A comprehensive health program among South African Zulus. In Paul BD (ed): Health, Culture and Community. New York, Russell Sage Foundation, 1955.

82. Lambo AT: Traditional African cultures and western medicine. A critical review. In Poynter FNL (ed): Medicine and Culture. London, Wellcome Institute of the History of Medicine, 1969, p 201.

83. ———: The village of Aro. In King M (ed): Medical Care in Developing Countries. London, Oxford Univ. Press, 1966, chap 20.

84. Conco WZ: The African Bantu traditional practice of medicine: some preliminary observations. Soc Sci Med 6:283, 1972.

85. Evans-Pritchard EE: Witchcraft, Oracles and Magic among the Azande. London, Oxford Univ. Press, 1937.

86. Bannerman RHO, Cummins A, Djukanovic V, et al.: Indigenous systems of medicine: Ayuverdic medicine in India. In Djukanovic V, Mach EP (eds): Alternative Approaches to Meeting Basic Health Needs in Developing Countries. Geneva, WHO, 1975, p 84.
87. Smith AJ: Best of the old and the new. Br Med J 2:367, 1974.
88. Sidel VW: The role and training of medical personnel. In Wegman ME, Tsung-yi Lin, Purcell EF (eds): Public Health in the People's Republic of China. New York, Josiah Macy Foundation, 1973, p 158.
89. Sidel VW, Sidel R: Serve the People. Observations on Medicine in the People's Republic of China. New York, Josiah Macy Foundation, 1973.
90. Wilenski P: The Delivery of Health Services in the People's Republic of China. Ottawa, International Development Research Centre, 1976.

CHAPTER 4

COMMUNITY HEALTH CARE
IN AN URBAN NEIGHBORHOOD

Rapid urban development is a worldwide phenomenon involving many millions of people and presenting difficult challenges to health and welfare services, to education and housing, and to community organization. In some cities, the large number of immigrants differ not only from the old-timers but from one another in culture and language, race and religion, to the point where there is no obvious sense of community or belonging. Sometimes, there is not only a lack of communication between people living on the same street, or even in the same high-rise building, but mutual suspicion and fear pervade the neighborhood. The newcomers may have migrated from other parts of the country itself or from other countries, and reaction of the settled population is often evidenced in behavior ranging from mild joking at the expense of the immigrants to extreme forms of hostile reaction with the formation of racist political parties.

Natural boundaries of the neighborhood community are not always readily obvious, as they are in rural villages or in well-established cities, some of which have grown almost by the fusion of preexisting villages. Such are many of the older cities of the world.

A community-based and community-oriented health care center in such circumstances is fraught with many serious challenges, not the least of which is the highly mobile and "noncommunity" nature of the population. The high mobility of people is an obstacle to the development of continuity in practitioner-patient relationships and long-term community health programs. Such populations also often have distinctive demographic features. Young migrant male workers, teenage and young adult women, often constitute a large proportion of the population. Other social selective processes result in many city centers having a high concentration of maladjusted individuals with mental disease and social pathology, such as drug addiction and alcoholism.

Yet another problem facing the establishment of community health care in urban neighborhoods is the nature and extent of existing services. There is often a plethora of different services, controlled by various agencies with their vested interests and commitments. Usually uncoordinated, they are used frequently and often ineffectively by the people. It is in these circumstances that emergency rooms and outpatient departments of hospitals become major centers for general primary care, often resulting in an impersonal, relatively anonymous type of health care. This is a highly selective phenomenon, frequently involving the poor, immigrants and newcomers, and the socially maladjusted of many cities. It is a sad and distressing feature of modern health care in the rapidly growing cities of many developed and developing countries, and is a reflection of society's failure to recognize the importance of community-oriented primary care, which might help meet the social, mental, and physical health needs of these populations.

Many models of community health centers have evolved in rural village communities or small towns, with their relatively stable populations. In these circumstances, the possibility of applying modern concepts of integrated health services is tempting, and is in fact relatively simple. However, these models are not necessarily applicable to the growing modern city, with its teeming heterogeneous masses of people. There are some who go so far as to say that the orientation of such health centers is neither suitable nor possible in these urban populations. Nevertheless, the contribution of community-oriented primary health care to community development and health in these settings needs serious consideration.

Health services may fulfill social functions beyond those they intend or for which they are recognized. Thus, like other institutions, they may have latent functions they do not profess to practice.[1] This was illustrated by Shuval and her associates in a study of the social functions of medical practice, which involved investigation of clinic utilization by different groups of immigrants to Israel after the establishment of the state in 1948.[2] They found an association between clinic utilization and immigration. Those who had not yet entered fully into the mainstream of Israeli life had a relatively high frequency of utilization. This may in itself be associated with higher rates of illness, but their findings indicate a utilization of clinic services beyond commonly recognized medical needs; these included the need for catharsis and help in coping with failure. These needs are common to populations other than immigrants, and are no doubt a factor in people turning toward doctors as patients. Meeting such psychosocial needs should be a more explicit function in the practice of family and community health care.

While mobility is a feature of many urban neighborhoods, closer examination may indicate that considerable numbers of families are long-term residents; they constitute a stable core with well-knit networks of relationships involving kin, friends, and other groups in the neighborhood and beyond. Furthermore, mobility is a selective process in which such factors as age are important. Younger adults, with or without children, tend to have much higher rates than the middle-aged and elderly. It is important to appreciate that mobility in itself is not synonymous either with the absence of meaningful relationships nor with social disorganization. People often form groups with common interests, such as "staircase communities" in high-rise buildings, mothers of young children, and neighbors. Both well-knit, solidary groups and more loosely knit networks of relationships are to be found in cities.[3-5] They are an important part of the supportive system of individuals and families and hence are potentially significant resources in community health care.

Even in the least promising setting, where social disorganization may be most evident, an explicitly stated objective of community-oriented primary health care should be the encouragement of social supportive systems for mutual health care. In this way, relating individuals, be they kin, neighbors, or friends, may be helped to develop reciprocal functions in times of illness, disability, or other crisis situations. This strengthens the case for community-based and socially oriented health care.

A COMMUNITY-ORIENTED NEIGHBORHOOD HEALTH CENTER IN JERUSALEM

It was in such an urban setting that the community health center to be described was established in 1953 by the Hadassah Medical Organization.[6,7] This center is situated in Kiryat Yovel, a western area of Jerusalem. The neighborhood began as an urban development project in which many thousands of immigrant families, and lesser numbers of Israel-born and earlier immigrants, settled since its inception in 1951. It now has a population exceeding 25,000.

There is a wide range of housing. Buildings of two stories with four to eight apartments predominate, and single-family homes on their own plots are also to be found. Larger multistoried units have been built, and the density of population in the neighborhood is increasing. It has some of the finest houses in Jerusalem, built along the hills overlooking the valleys below to the historic village of Ein Karem. Here also, until very recently, were some of the worst homes of Jerusalem, in which lived relatively poor and uneducated families. The houses were temporary structures built of asbestos, spread across a whole valley of the area. As families are rehoused in other parts of the city, these temporary houses are being demolished.

It is a growing area of a city, itself becoming a bustling, active capital of the country. It is traversed by roads that link various parts of the neighborhood with the city center, through which buses and other traffic also pass beyond Kiryat Yovel to still more distant areas of the city. Shopping centers, schools, a variety of public services, university student residences, and a reception center for new immigrants all add to the setting of this district of Jerusalem. Situated a few kilometers further west is the large Hadassah-Hebrew University medical center, with its hospital, medical, nursing, dental, pharmacy, and public health schools.

In 1951, Kiryat Yovel was not yet incorporated into Jerusalem. It lay to the west of the growing city, a sparsely populated area on the urban periphery. It was then that the first of the new housing projects was built. The need for settlement of immigrants was very great, with the result that immigrant families were settled in them before they were completed and before roads and transportation had been properly developed.

At the time the health center commenced its activities, in January 1953, the diversity of ethnic groups was a striking feature of the neighborhood. Families originating from more than 25 countries were settled in the first immigrant housing project, and neighbors had very limited communication. In many buildings, there were families from several countries, with different languages, culture, and behavior. The present social class differences of neighborhoods within the area were already evident then. There were different housing projects, one for new immigrants, another for veteran trade union members, and yet another for public servants centered in Jerusalem. The projects housing these groups were readily distinguishable. Not only was each project geographically defined, but the social distance was readily observed by the general appearance of the homes, the state of their immediate environs, and the kind and standard of dress of adults and children. These differences are still evident, although considerably less marked.

The Health and Welfare Services of Jerusalem

When the health center was established, the health services of Jerusalem were conducted by separate agencies having little, if any, accountability to one another or to a central authority. There was some interaction in the care of individual patients, but there was no organization for coordinating the functions of the various agencies involved, nor was there a strong central authority. The Ministry of Health had itself only recently been established and, as with other fields of public administration, it lacked experienced public health personnel.

There are two distinct, and separately provided, forms of community-based personal health services in Jerusalem, preventive and curative. This reflects the situation in the country as a whole, except for the spread of centers such as the community health center in Kiryat Yovel. The preventive services in Jerusalem consist mostly of maternal and child health centers and school health services, both conducted by the health department of the city. Community-based curative services are provided for the most part by clinics, established in various parts of the city by the Sick Fund of the National Federation of Labor Unions (Kupat Holim). Welfare services are provided independently of both these services by the Family and Community Welfare Department of the city, except that the Ministry of Welfare has an arrangement whereby Kupat Holim provides for the curative care of persons and families "on welfare." The three services, preventive, curative, and welfare, are separately housed.

In regard to hospital care, all the general hospitals of Jerusalem are conducted by non-profit voluntary organizations. This is unlike the situation in other major cities of the country, where the Ministry of Health, municipal authority, or the Kupat Holim are responsible for the major hospitals. Through its two Jerusalem hospitals, at Ein Karem and on Mount Scopus, Hadassah has over 1000 beds and also provides emergency and extensive outpatient specialist services.

Health Care in Kiryat Yovel

The health facilities available to the people of Kiryat Yovel are much the same as those described for Jerusalem as a whole. Both curative and preventive clinics are situated in various parts of the area, within relatively easy walking distance of most homes. With the exception of our departmental health center, the curative and preventive clinics are separately housed and administered. In addition, the welfare services in the area are the responsibility of a special department of the municipality and are located separately from the health services.

It is well accepted that continuity of care is in the interests of the well and the sick, of families and their individual members. However, the health services of Jerusalem, and in Kiryat Yovel itself, do not encourage continuity of care. As residents of Jerusalem, with transportation readily available to various parts of the city, the people of Kiryat Yovel have access to, and use, various health services in the city. In a setting in which there are a multiplicity of agencies offering individual care in different institutions, there is likely to be much overlap and discontinuity in the services a patient receives. There are also likely to be gaps in care and limited continuity of care in the full meaning of the term. Patients are attended by different physicians, who are not usually members of the same team. There may also be discontinuity of care for patients needing repeated hospitalization, as they are sometimes admitted to different hospitals for recurrent episodes of a single illness. One of the aims of our health center is to reduce the sense of discontinuity of care felt by patients, by maintaining contact with them and their families, and, where necessary, providing treatment and home care regardless of the particular clinic, emergency service, or hospital attended by the patient.

Some unsatisfactory aspects of a nonunified health care system are:

Problems created by the ready access to so many varied health and medical care facilities.
The limited relationship between the various services.
The absence of responsibility by any single agency for the overall health of a person, or of families and the community.

With the possible exception of the citywide maternal and child health services, a main feature of the personal services is that the initiative for care only comes from patient or family. The service does not go out into the community, exploring and investigating health problems and initiating care. In contrast to this static type of service is that of public health, in which mobility is a feature. This is one of the main aspects of our health center's approach, namely, going out to the community to conduct investigations into its health, health attitudes, and health-relevant practices. On the basis of the findings, action is initiated by the health center. All this is done with the concurrence of the community and its increasing participation.

THE PRESENT-DAY PRACTICE
OF THE HEALTH CENTER

The health center is now an integral part of the department of social medicine of the Hebrew University-Hadassah Medical School, in much the same way as the wards of the teaching hospitals are functions of various clinical departments of its medical and nursing schools. We have focused the present-day practice of the department of social medicine in Kiryat Yovel on the development of a unified practice of community medicine and primary health care. We are doing this in several different kinds of practices conducted from the health center, including a general family practice, maternal and child health care, and home care of housebound patients. Recently, the department of child psychiatry of the Hadassah hospital has initiated a child and family psychiatric practice in our health center. Its area of practice in Kiryat Yovel is the same as that defined for child health care by the health center. Ways of working together are being actively explored.

Changes that have been made in the practice of the health center result from its experience over the 28 years since its inception, changes in Kiryat Yovel itself, the growth of Jerusalem and its health services, and the development of the center's role in the teaching and demonstration functions of the university department of social medicine.

The Family Practice of the Health Center

The family practice provides comprehensive health care to approximately 1000 families, comprising over 3000 people, of whom some 2000 live in a defined geographic area of Kiryat Yovel. This area consists of the original housing projects built for new immigrants in 1951. The first inhabitants came from various countries of North Africa, the Middle East, Europe, and the Americas. It was to these families that much attention was initially given, based on the decision that the health center should aim to assist in the process of assimilating an immigrant population.

A considerable proportion of the younger adults, and almost all the children now living there, were born in Israel, and the age structure of the population included in the family practice has changed considerably. While in 1956 less than 5 percent of the population registered in this practice were 65 years of age or older, in 1977 they constituted more than 12 percent of the family practice population living in the original housing projects. This is well above the corresponding figure for Kiryat Yovel as a whole and is related to selective emigration from these homes by younger adults with their families. With increase in age of the population, another striking fact has emerged, namely, 23 percent of the homes are inhabited by one person only, usually aged. More than one in every four of the older population (65 years and over) is homebound, and these people constitute almost 80 percent of all cases being cared for by the health center's home care service.

In the early years of the health center, the health team gave much attention to the health problems of young families, with emphasis on maternal and child health care. While this group is obviously still important and receives considerable attention, there has been an important shift in the focus of the practice to concern with the health needs of the growing proportion of aged persons.

The family practice is a community-oriented primary health care service, combining care of individual patients and families with that of the community as a whole. In so doing, it is a unified promotive, preventive, and curative practice. Generally, a family practice is essentially a service in response to patients who turn to it for care or advice. However, as the community-oriented programs develop there is an increasing degree of initiative by the family practice in arranging for appointments with doctors and nurses. In a primary-care practice, reaching out to the community involves contact with individuals and families. It is important to stress the change from traditional medical care that this brings about. Instead of being confined to situations in which patients seek a service and the doctor or nurse responds to the demand, it expands to one in which the community eventually becomes increasingly participant in meeting its own needs.

The Daily Activities of the Family Physicians and Nurses.
Clinics. The day begins with clinics receiving patients of any age, seeking care wihout prior appointment. These may be people with acute illness, exacerbations of chronic conditions, worries, or other problems they feel to be urgent. The early mornings in the family practice thus present a busy scene. There are similar clinics later in the day, or early evenings, for the convenience of workers and others.

Apart from these daily clinics there are a number of different activities:

>   Appointments with patients, which are initiated by patients themselves, nurses, or doctors. These may be any one of the many chronic sick patients, with physical or mental conditions, or family members about a patient or a personal family problem.
>
>   Special sessions for those in community health programs, such as the community cardiovascular disease and diabetes program (CHAD), which includes all adults in the population; maternal and child health sessions for expectant mothers, postnatal examinations and family planning, and well babies.

Home Visits.   These constitute a very significant part of the family nurses' activities, for care of the sick and disabled, for surveillance and health education of families with mothers and babies, older people, persons living alone, and for various other family problems. The family physicians conduct daily rounds of patients at home, usually at the request of the family nurse or the family itself.

Visits to Schools.   Doctors and nurses of the family practice visit the nursery schools and schools of the area as part of the school health program.

Conferences and Teaching.   In addition to frequent informal case discussions during the course of the day, there are meetings of various kinds. These include administrative staff meetings, doctors' clinical conferences, weekly community medicine program reviews, special teaching sessions, meetings with the community health council, and other activities.

During a year, 1976, the family practice cared for 3287 individuals, with a total of 14,240 contacts with physicians of the practice. The average of 4.3 contacts per person for both curative and preventive care is a relatively low figure for urban areas in Israel, well below half the average attendance at the curative primary-care clinics of the country. If one were to add to the latter the contacts made at the separate preventive clinics conducted in the country, the disparity would be even greater. We believe that the cause of this favorable trend toward a more balanced utilization of primary-care facilities is a result of the particular approach of this practice. Among the outstanding features is the doctor-nurse team combining curative and preventive functions, providing for continuity of care of individuals in the framework of a family- and community-oriented practice.

Maternal and Child Health Care

This includes:

Care of expectant and postnatal mothers.
Well babies and toddlers.
Schoolchildren, including nursery schools, kindergartens, and elementary schools.

In addition to the maternal and child health care provided by the family practice for its defined population, the health center is responsible for maternal and child health care for the population of other neighborhood communities in Kiryat Yovel. Unlike the family practice, these maternal and child health services provide promotive and preventive care only, and are thus more in line with the traditional maternal and child health services in this country and many others. The major difference in these services from those of other parts of the country is in the development of problem-oriented community medicine intervention programs.

Specially prepared guides for the team outline the routine care of mothers and babies. They include details of the number and time of examinations to be performed by physicians and by nurses, the content of these examinations, and intervention, such as immunizations. These are updated to incorporate recent advances, for example, testing for rubella antibodies in pregnancy and referral for possible amniocentesis.

Between 300 and 400 births are registered annually in these communities, and 95 to 100 percent of mothers use the facilities at the center for their babies. More than 80 percent of mothers who give birth attend the health center for their prenatal care. A gynecologist-obstetrician participates in this at the health center by conducting at least one prenatal examination and postnatal examinations.

School Health Services. As already indicated, the health center also has responsibilities for several schools and kindergartens in the Kiryat Yovel community. The physicians and nurses of the health center have a well-established procedure of case discussions and consultations with child psychiatrists based at the health center, school psychologists, and social workers. In this way, a widely based perspective of the problems of numbers of children is ensured. The schoolteachers themselves are involved in these reviews; more than 600 sessions are held in the course of a year. The four elementary schools for which the center has these responsibilities have over 2000 children, and there are approximately 600 children in kindergartens. The greatest part of this preventive service for the children and their parents is carried out by the public health nurses of the health center with the pediatricians and family physicians. Among the activities are initial health examinations, vision and hearing tests, immunizations, and health education, including sex education.

Home Care Service of Homebound Patients

In addition to the treatment of patients at home, which has been undertaken for those patients cared for by the family practice since its inception, an expanded service covering the needs of homebound patients was established in 1966. Those served include homebound patients living in any part of Kiryat Yovel, with its population of about 25,000. There are approximately 130 patients under care at any time, and when necessary, the services of a physiotherapist, an occupational therapist, and consultations with social workers are obtained. Many of these patients also receive home-help services and feeding through "meals on wheels."

Laboratory and Pharmacy

The health center laboratory undertakes a considerable number of examinations, in addition to those sent to the more specialized laboratories of the hospital. It is of advantage to the health team, and of considerable convenience to the community, to have a laboratory located in the health center.

The pharmacy is another service for the convenience of patients, and it can act as an important health education instrument by the pharmacist's explanations to patients about drugs, their storage, precautions needed, and compliance.

Before more detailed consideration of community medicine in the primary health care of the health center, it is useful to summarize the various types of primary care for individuals provided by the several practices of the health center. Thus, in the family practice, there is a unified preventive and curative service for all who are registered with it; in the separate maternal and child health clinics the service is promotive and preventive, the curative aspects being provided by other agencies; in the home care service, curative and rehabilitative care is provided to disabled homebound patients. These differences in care of individual patients provide the opportunity for experience with differing ways of delivering health care in the community, whether at the clinics of the health center, in patients' homes, or at schools.

COMMUNITY MEDICINE IN PRIMARY CARE

The community health care activities of the health center include orientation toward the community as a whole or its subgroups as well as to individual patients and their families. The community and individual care is provided in the framework of the following primary care units of the center:

> General family practice.
> Maternal and child health clinics.
> School health service.
> Home care.

The development of community medicine within the framework of such different primary health care practices needs new health teams, including primary-care physicians and nurses, epidemiologists and biostatisticians, and special personnel concerned with health-related behavior, health education and community organization. Several such teams function in the health center, together constituting a group having the common objective of developing community-oriented care in different types of primary health practices. Community-oriented health care and its incorporation into the family practice of the health center will be discussed further.

Community Medicine in Family Practice.   In combining community medicine with the primary health care of individuals in the family practice of this health center, it must be noted that this practice differs from the usual personal health care in Israel in three major respects:

1. It combines curative and preventive services within a single practice, provided by a team of physicians, nurses, and a community organizer/health educator.
2. It uses epidemiologic concepts and methods in developing a community orientation within the primary health care of the practice.
3. The community is becoming increasingly involved in the functioning of the health center, both in active participation of community members in decision making and in various activities.

Figure 4-1 represents the way curative and preventive clinics have been combined in the family practice, with the subsequent development of community medicine using epidemiologic skills.

Community medicine intervention programs may also be developed within the framework of separate curative clinics or preventive services. We have done this extensively in the preventive maternal and child health unit of the health center, and, in collaboration with the city health department, are extending it to other such units in Jerusalem.

Planning a Community Program.   Initiating a community program within a primary-care practice requires careful consideration, as it demands much from the health team and the community. The initial case for planning such a program depends on a number of factors, such as:

Clinical impressions of the extent and importance of the problem in the particular population, supported by evidence of its prevalence in the wider region of which the community is a part.

The possibility that intervention will be acceptable to the community and can be expected to have an effective outcome.

The feasibility of carrying out a suitable community health program in the framework of primary care.

Planning of various programs requires decision on priorities in the practice, which will be determined by the preceding considerations and the skills, interests, and motivation of different members of the health team. In order to use such a primary-care health center as an instrument of public health to improve the community's health, the planning of various community health programs has included:

Ways of gathering information, its recording and analysis, for community diagnosis of health conditions and their determinants, and what is already being done about them.

A program of action focused on target groups and aiming to ensure satisfactory response from all the individuals and the community groups concerned.

Ways of continuing surveillance of the health condition itself, and the extent to which the planned program is being achieved.

Methods of evaluation of the program, with special reference to its effectiveness.

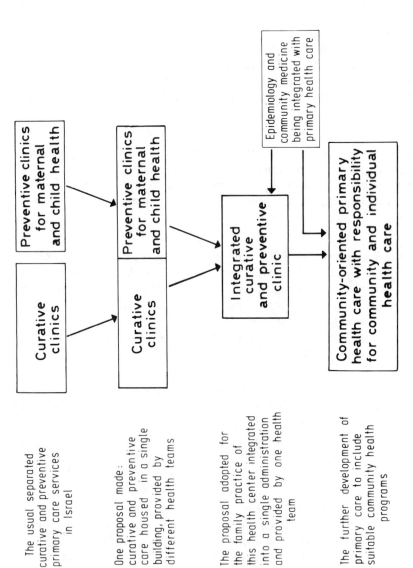

FIG. 4-1. Steps in integrating community medicine into a primary health center.

The usual separated curative and preventive primary care services in Israel

One proposal made: curative and preventive care housed in a single building, provided by different health teams

The proposal adopted for the family practice of this health center integrated into a single administration and provided by one health team

The further development of primary care to include suitable community health programs

Preventive clinics for maternal and child health

Curative clinics

Preventive clinics for maternal and child health

Curative clinics

Integrated curative and preventive clinic

Epidemiology and community medicine being integrated with primary health care

Community-oriented primary health care with responsibility for community and individual health care

THE COMMUNITY MEDICINE PROGRAMS

The existing community medicine programs include those focused on the population as a whole:

Surveillance of demographic changes in the community.
Surveys of the community's health for health surveillance, intervention, and evaluation.
Surveillance and control of communicable disease.

and on three broad phases of life:

Reproduction and family formation.
Childhood from infancy through adolescence.
Adulthood from young adult through to the elderly and aged.

The Population as a Whole

Surveillance of Demographic Changes in the Community.   There have been marked demographic changes in this community, first through settlement of new families, as well as out-migration, births, and deaths. Records of all births and deaths are maintained in the health center. Official sources of notification are matched with information obtained from hospitals and personal information to the nurses and doctors from families in the community. Estimates of population are made from intercensal data prepared by the Israel Bureau of Statistics and community surveys conducted by the health center.

This allows for periodic analysis and review of birth and death rates, causes of death, and important demographic and social changes in the population. The changes have included increase in the standards of education of men, women, and children, in the age distribution toward an older population, and in the ethnic group distribution. All these are taken into account in planning new community health programs or modifying ongoing programs.

A difficulty in the pursuit of long-term community health programs is the mobility of a population. In fact, this is often used as an argument against the feasibility of such programs in city areas. However, each community needs careful study of this phenomenon, as there may be differences in the mobility of different segments of the population. This was analyzed in two statistical census tracts of Kiryat Yovel. The average annual total mobility rate over a 3-year period was 13.2 percent in an estimated population of 4100. Children and young adults, aged below 30 years, constituted between 75 and 80 percent of all inward and outward movements of these areas, with the out movements exceeding movements into the areas by an average of more than 4 percent per year. This disparity was especially marked for children below 15 years, where the ratio of out- to in-movements was greater than 5 to 1. Our community programs focused on child development and growth have been considerably affected by this process, much more so than the programs concerned with older people.

In the same area, the annual average birth rate was 30 per 1000 population, and the crude mortality rate was 9.3. Despite these figures, the population is aging, a fact resulting from the selective process of emigration of families with young children from the area.

Surveys of the Community's Health for Health Surveillance, Intervention, and Evaluation

Two general community health surveys have been completed. The first, which commenced in late 1969 and continued through to middle 1971, included approximately 10,000 people.[8,9] This was designed to be a study of a total population along the lines of the Tecumseh total community health study.[10] Planned and carried out as an epidemiologic research project, it was also a foundation for community diagnosis and a controlled intervention trial. This was possible because the population of the community health survey included those living in the geographic area of the family practice as well as those in contiguous parts of Kiryat Yovel, who receive their general curative service from other agencies.

With the baseline knowledge provided by this first comprehensive community health survey, a second health survey was conducted 5 years later (1975 to 1976). This was less comprehensive, confined to the adult population, and focused especially on the circulatory system. It allowed for measurement of changes in the health status of the population in the 5-year period since the first survey and for evaluation of some aspects of the CHAD community medicine intervention program.

A third round is being planned to commence in 1980. It is hoped that this survey will be conducted as a regular part of the family practice, as periodic health examinations of the adult population in the practice. The control population will also be examined, but no longer as a control group, since the clinic that provides for their curative care has invited staff of the health center to assist it in developing a community health program, concerned with hypertension in the first instance.

Surveillance and Control of Communicable Disease. The surveillance is part of a system of monitoring all contacts the family physicians have with patients. Each doctor in the family practice has a set of specially prepared contact sheets on the consulting room desk. One is completed for each patient seen, and every day the chief family physician, together with a health recorder, extracts information on the cases with infectious diseases. The data are charted by day of onset and by disease on a wall chart in the health center. This kind of recording of communicable disease was first used by Pickles of Yorkshire, England, in his rural general practice.[11] Analysis of the accumulated data is reported, showing trends of infectious disease in the community.[12]

The program includes immunizations for the total community of children as part of the maternal and child health service. The immunizations are: oral polio, triple vaccine (diphtheria, pertussis, and tetanus), and measles; smallpox vaccination is no longer required. Immunization against rubella is done in all 12-year-old girls at school and in postpartum women, if negative for antibodies during pregnancy. In addition, elderly persons and patients at risk are offered immunization against influenza before winter each year.

At one time, the health center had a special program for the prevention and control of rheumatic fever and rheumatic heart disease. It continued over a period of some 15 years (1959 to the mid-1970s). For a number of years there were no new cases, which reflected a dramatic decline of the disease in Jerusalem and the country as a whole. Therefore, the community program was terminated, while routine prophylaxis of the known cases continued.[13]

Reproduction and Family Formation

The main community programs carried out by the health center, in respect of the health aspects of reproduction and family formation, are those concerning pregnancy and its outcome and family planning.

Pregnancy and Its Outcome. Pre- and postnatal care of mothers and their babies is associated with health surveillance, the 28th-day program, in which a record is accumulated of the condition of mothers through pregnancy, the delivery and puerperium, and of their babies' state at birth, through the neonatal period, and at the 28th-day examination. Associated with this health surveillance, specific community health programs are developed; these include the control of anemia in pregnancy and the treatment of asymptomatic bacteriuria.[14] Some aspects of this subject are discussed in more detail in Chapter 5.

Family Planning. This has included surveys of mothers' attitudes as to the desired size of family, spacing between children, and contraceptive practices. The center has developed a program of advice, prescription, and the fitting of suitable contraceptives. It is now a routine part of postnatal care provided by the center.

The use of contraceptives by postnatal women changed considerably through the 1970s. In two studies of postnatal women attending the health center, 148 in 1971 and 188 in 1977, the proportion using the pill, IUD, or condom increased from 33 to 62 percent, and the numbers using the safe period or coitus interruptus declined from 60 to 25 percent over this 6-year period. The family practice and maternal and child health service of the center are now developing the family planning service as a well-defined community program. The decision to do this follows on the evidence of a desire for such a program by the people who are eligible to use the health center's primary-care services.

Childhood from Infancy Through Adolescence

The main community medicine program for this category is focused on the promotion of child growth and development (PROD). It includes community diagnosis of physical growth, behavior, and intellectual development, anemia in infancy, infectious diseases, and other illnesses that might affect growth. The community diagnosis guides us to the type of intervention likely to be most effective. The program has been designed to focus on the key family risk factors associated with the level of development of infants and young children in this community, from birth through to 5 years of age. The surveillance is associated with special programs, over and above the already highly developed system of well-child care in the country. The program is outlined in more detail in Chapter 5.

The school health service of the health center, outlined earlier, is being developed to include several community health programs. Among these is one concerning learning disabilities, organized by the department of child psychiatry in association with the health center and the schools in Kiryat Yovel. A reevaluation of other routines is also being undertaken, with the differences in vision and hearing being analyzed for various groups of children, including social class differences.

Adulthood and Aging

The major public health problem is a community syndrome of coronary heart disease, cerebral vascular disease, hypertension, hypercholesterolemia, and diabetes. We have, therefore, developed an intervention program concerned with surveillance and control of a number of factors associated with high risk for these diseases. We refer to this as a program for the control of the community syndrome of *h*ypertension, *a*therosclerotic diseases, and *d*iabetes (CHAD). This is described in Chapter 6.

COMMUNITY PARTICIPATION
IN THE HEALTH CENTER'S ACTIVITIES

Community involvement in the conduct of health services has not been a feature of urban neighborhoods in the country. The public's involvement in health care is mainly at the level of central and local authority government. Until recently, Kiryat Yovel did not differ from other neighborhoods in this respect. However, for many years there have been close relationships between staff of the health center and members of the community. Community participation in the health center's activities was mainly in utilization of the services and response to surveys and programs initiated by the center.

There was a lack of community participation in the planning and decision-making aspects of the center and in actual involvement in providing health care. There had been encouraging developments of this kind, including the formation of a diabetic group and an old-age club, but these did not involve the community as a whole.

An opportunity for more comprehensive and active involvement of the community occurred during the twenty-fifth anniversary celebrations of the health center. Members of the community decided to host a festive evening for the center, for which they prepared a variety of traditional dishes for a dinner, followed by speeches, folk dancing, and stage performances by various groups of the community. The theme of the evening was the history of the community, with its varied ethnic origins, and their experiences with the health center. The warm feelings expressed about the center and its team were an outstanding feature of the evening.

Many members of the community were clearly very able, sophisticated organizers, who were closely identified with the health center and obviously ready to become more involved. It was then decided that the time was ripe to initiate more organized and active community participation. This began with a meeting at the health center of a group consisting of members of the community and representatives of several agencies in the community, including the health center. The group decided to form an organization for coordinating health, welfare, and educational activities in Kiryat Yovel.

The membership includes community members, elected by the local Kiryat Yovel community council, representatives of the health center and other health agencies in the area, and representatives of the area community centers, schools, synagogues, and welfare agencies.

Several working groups were formed to deal with different health and welfare activities, such as the group to undertake organization of a supportive program of visits and aid by community members to homebound and disabled patients. Another group consists of representatives of the health center's family practice team and the families eligible to use this service. The immediate purpose is for the community members to be an advisory group to the health center, and eventually to develop into a joint planning and decision-making group.

These activities are a beginning of an important process in community participation in the promotion of their health and welfare.

COMMUNITY MEDICINE ROUNDS (CMR)

The different practices of the health center are reviewed at regular weekly conferences. These are the nearest approach we have to the grand rounds and clinical pathologic conferences of teaching hospitals. They involve review and evaluation of progress of the health center practices, the various community medicine programs in these practices, together with demographic and epidemiologic reports.

At these conferences, one of the central questions concerns the role of epidemiology in uniting community medicine and primary health care. Its functions become more defined in our exploration of problems in community diagnosis, continuing surveillance of health and health care, and evaluation of the programs. We are concerned not only with epidemiologic research in a family practice or other type of primary health care, but also with the use of epidemiology as an essential instrument in promoting a fresh approach to health care, namely, community-oriented primary health care. The various health teams, consisting of faculty members of the department and staff of the health center, participate in this weekly review: It is thus a meeting of minds of different professional groups, epidemiologists and clinicians, physicians, nurses, community health workers, health statisticians, and health recorders.

The CMR is held at the health center in a conference room in which data of ongoing activities are charted on the walls as visual aids. The individual participants, and especially the health teams, have an active role in these sessions. Each health team has the responsibility of reviewing the progress of its work at least once during the year, and usually more often. The frequency depends on the development of the program. Thus, in a community program aimed to maintain surveillance of hemoglobin levels and treatment of anemia during pregnancy, the frequency of review has declined from once weekly to once annually, as the amount of anemia has declined. Similarly, with programs such as that concerned with prophylaxis of rheumatic fever and rheumatic heart disease, and with immunizations, an annual review, or even less often, suffices.

On the other hand, frequent reviews are made of community programs such as those concerned with pregnancy and its outcome, the promotion of growth and development of infants and children, and the control and prevention of cardiovascular and cerebrovascular diseases.

Recently, we have included reviews of programs in which departmental members are engaged at other centers, in Jerusalem and other parts of the country. Thus in the past year several new programs have been reviewed. They have included:

The utilization of primary health care facilities in several localities, namely, northeast Jerusalem, the town of Ashkelon, and a number of rural villages in Jerusalem district. These have been joint staff-student projects.

Case finding and treatment of hypertension by Kupat Holim clinics in Jerusalem. The programs are the responsibility of different groups. Thus, the program in one clinic of northeast Jerusalem is the responsibility of the department of internal medicine of the Hadassah hospital on Mount Scopus, together with members of our department and the local community.

One of the objectives of the CMR is that each participant has an active role to fulfill in these sessions and is concerned with one or more aspects of the community's health and the action being taken. The topics to be reviewed are decided upon by the conference group, and a revised schedule is prepared for each year. Reviews of well-established programs are a main feature of the CMR, but another important function is consideration of proposals for new programs. Surveillance of health of the populations involved in the various primary health care services has been steadily extended and, as the need arises, a new community medicine program is prepared.

This is a useful teaching session, at which medical students and postgraduate public health students are present. They may participate in presentation of a topic together with team members, or they may present their own community-oriented studies.

Examples of community-oriented primary health care programs

reviewed in weekly conferences, CMR, at the health center in Kiryat Yovel:

Demography of the practice populations:
Births and deaths, birth rates and mortality rates.
Population change: age, sex, ethnic group, and family size.

Infectious illnesses:
Review of all acute infectious illnesses diagnosed in the family practice and immunization programs of the health center.

The 28th-day review:
This includes a review of all pregnancies and births, as normal or abnormal in pregnancy, labor, child at birth, and neonatal period to 28th day.
Report on action programs and investigations:
Anemia in pregnancy.
Smoking in pregnancy.
Family spacing in the postnatal program.

Promotion of growth and development during infancy and childhood (PROD):
Cumulative measurement of growth and development trends, including:
Physical growth, behavior development, intellectual development (IQ).
Reports on action programs and investigations:
Feeding practices.
Anemia in infancy.
Infections in infancy.
Verbal and social stimulation.

Other child health programs:
School surveys of hearing and vision.
Chronic disease and disability in children.

Community program for control and treatment of hypertension, hyperlipidemia, diabetes mellitus, coronary heart disease, and cerebrovascular disease (CHAD):
Reports on action programs and investigations:
Risk factors and diseases:
Blood pressure and hypertension.
Serum lipids and hypercholesterolemia.
Diabetes mellitus.
Ischemic heart disease, cerebrovascular disease, and peripheral vascular disease.

Behavior-related factors:
Diet, exercise, smoking, use of services, and response to the program.
Facilities for change and treatment:
CHAD clinics, community organization, and health education.

Home care:
Review of program.

Health care:
Surveys and reviews of utilization and satisfaction with primary health care in various localities.
Perceptions of health in different communities.
Community participation, reports on progress.

THE HEALTH TEAM

The development of community medicine within a family practice or health center requires bringing together different skills represented by primary-care physicians and nurses, epidemiologists, and biostatisticians, as well as professionals concerned with health-related behavior, health education, and community organization. As an example, we will consider the family practice team of the health center. The team responsible for this practice at the present time consists of the following members:

Family physicians and family nurses.
Members with special skills in community medicine, namely, epidemiology, biostatistics, community organization, and health education.
Consultants, such as in pediatrics, internal medicine, nutrition, psychiatry, gynecology, and others.
Supportive members of the team. Administration, secretarial assistance, health records, laboratory, and pharmacy.

The Family Physicians and Family Nurses

From its inception in 1953, a distinctive feature of the health center's family practice has been the allotment of a neighborhood of homes to a team of family doctors and nurses. The objective was that the same doctors and nurses attended to individuals and families during health and illness.

Two physicians and four nurses constitute the core group of the family practice, being the key persons involved in day-to-day contact with patients and families, each nurse having responsibility for an area and two nurses working with each of the doctors. The complementary roles of doctors and nurses involve both professional groups in curative as well as preventive work.

Except for newcomers to the area, today there are very few people in the community who have not previously been seen by at least one team member. Stability of staff members has been an outstanding feature of the team. Of the two senior family physicians, one has been in this practice since its beginning in 1953 and the other since 1964, and several of the nurses have also been in the practice for as much as 15 to 20 years. Mobility of population has been greater than that of doctors and nurses, but there is a core of families who have been in the practice for 20 years or more.

General curative work is carried out by the doctor-nurse team, at the clinic and at home. Depending on the reason for contact, patients may call at the center and be examined and treated at that time by their physician, or an appointment may be made for another occasion. Calls for home visits by doctor or nurse are made by telephone, by someone of the family coming to the center, or by the nurse asking the doctor to visit the home after she had visited there. With the change in age structure taking place in this community, and the increase in the number of aged people, care of the chronically ill is an important function of the team, including home care of housebound patients and aftercare of patients discharged from the hospital.

The preventive work has fully incorporated maternal and infant health care in the framework of the family practice. While special times are set aside for seeing well babies or pregnant women, they are seen by the same team members who would care for them when ill. Thus, the family nurse of this team is both a general curative nurse with skills in care and treatment at the clinic or at home, and a public health nurse with the ability to carry out a program for promoting health of expectant mothers and their infants and children. To be effective, this combination of curative, preventive, and promotive functions requires additional training of staff.

Combining curative and preventive functions by doctors and nurses in the care of their families is often considered to be a simple and easy task. A policy decision to do so is important, but it is only a beginning of a reeducation process, which involves widening the perception of their own roles and the learning of new skills.

In the earlier discussion of the family practice, the roles of the team's family physicians and nurses were considered, namely, in relation to individual and family care, without discussing details of their roles in the development of community medicine. This has been done for the sake of clarity in describing the changes needed in the team's role when initiating community medicine and primary health care as a unified practice. There is obviously a change in functions of a primary health care team when it extends its practice, from an orientation almost entirely focused on care of the individual in his family to a community-oriented practice in which community medicine and clinical practice are unified.

What are the skills doctors and nurses need in order to combine promotive, preventive, and curative functions in individual, family, and community health care?

1. *For Individual Care:*   The skills needed for integrating preventive and curative care of individuals include such procedures as:
   Clinical examination, diagnosis, and treatment of the sick patient.
   Measurement of growth and development of infants and children for the appraisal of physical growth, developmental diagnosis.
   Health examinations and interviews of children and adults, including pregnant and postnatal women, workers, elderly persons, and others.
   Screening examinations for case finding of important disorders.
   Ability to review findings with individual and family, and discuss desirable action. This involves health education and counseling regarding health-relevant behavior.

2. *For Family Health Care:*   The aspects considered here are:
   The family as a determinant of its individual members' health, and its care of well and sick individuals.
   Family diagnosis, that is, diagnosis of the state of health of the family as a group. This includes observation and description of patterns of health and disease; genetic, social, and environmental factors specific to a particular family; the implications for family health of its interaction with neighbors, kin, and others, and with the wider environment.
   Family consultation, discussing various findings and considering various action programs with the family.
   The family in community health. This includes consideration of the main family factors determining community health, such as genetic, reproduction and family formation, the psychosocial and biologic aspects of family structure and functioning.

3. *For Community Health Care:*   Methods of health examination of communities; the accumulation of data from various sources, including the case records of primary care practice; planning and con-

ducting surveys by household questionnaires and interviews, as well as clinical, somatometric, and psychologic examinations.

Community diagnosis and health surveillance as an integral part of primary health care, with emphasis on the use of epidemiology, biostatistics, and social science methods; initiating and using various types of community health registers; analysis of data, using computerized systems where possible.

Planning and implementing community medicine programs in primary care, including appropriate methods of evaluation.

Involvement of the community in its own health care.

4. *For the Development of a Doctor-Nurse Team in Community-Oriented Primary Health Care:*   The complementary functions of physicians and nurses need careful attention in the training program, since these health professionals have been educated apart from one another. As students, they seldom have the opportunity of learning about one another's functions, and what they may have had is usually restricted to a hospital setting. This creates several problems when they are brought together in a community-oriented primary health care practice. Physicians, while reorienting themselves in their new roles, need to modify their perceptions of the nurses' roles in this setting. Nurses need to do the same in respect to themselves and to physicians. In order to achieve this their training should be as members of a team in community-oriented primary care, having complementary roles. Before considering how this has been done, we need to discuss other members of the team.

Team Members with Special Skills in Community Medicine

Each community medicine program introduced into an ongoing primary-care practice of the health center has involved members of the department of social medicine who have special qualifications in fields such as epidemiology, biostatistics, community organization, or health education. Their roles range from consultants through to active participation in planning and carrying out various elements of the program for community diagnosis, intervention, community involvement, health surveillance, and program evaluation.

Community Organization and Health Education.   An important member of the team is a community organizer/health educator, who has had graduate training in both social work (community organization) and public health. One of the earliest objectives of the center was that of promoting community health, and since its inception it has been concerned with finding ways of doing this. Early on, the health center attempted to promote health through community action. While doctors, nurses, and other casework-oriented professional staff have a most important role in such community development work, the field extends beyond the main areas of experience of such personnel. The processes involved in community action concerned with the promotion of its own health are community organization and health education. Before the establishment of this health center, Israel had no experience with such personnel in health care. Despite this, it was agreed that the center should initiate a program of health education, and for this purpose several special appointments of community organizer/health educator were made to the health team.

In addition to the community organizer/health educator of the health center, the team has the support of several staff members of the department of social medicine, who are trained in one or more of the following: health education, community organization, psychology or one of the other behavioral sciences. Each has had further training to the master's or doctoral level in public health and social medicine. They function as consultants and supportive members of the health center team and participate in teaching programs conducted at the health center for its own staff and for students of the department. They also participate actively in various community health programs, including community surveys.

Epidemiology, Biostatistics, and Health Records. The epidemiology and biostatistics unit of the department of social medicine is actively involved in the community medicine programs developed by the health center. All proposed programs are considered by this unit together with the responsible primary-care team, the purpose being to ensure that they have sound epidemiologic foundations. Thus, members of the unit are involved as special members of the health center's team. All are now experienced in applying their skills to community-oriented primary health care.

The present chief of health records of the center is a graduate in statistics and has a master's degree in public health. She is a member of the epidemiology and biostatistics unit of the department, and teaches biostatistics as well as methods of health recording in community-oriented primary health care.

How Have Teams Been Trained To Fulfill the Roles Required in Community-Oriented Primary Health Care?

The process by which professional workers of different disciplines grow together as a team is complex, and the inevitability of gradual progress should be accepted. Providing that the difficulties, and the occasional failures, constitute a learning experience for those concerned with pioneering this approach to medical care, each difficulty will have served a useful function in testing various approaches.

Our early endeavors involved sensitizing the newly appointed staff of varying disciplines to the kinds of problems confronting them. This was done as an integral part of intensive in-service training of the team, in which different health-relevant beliefs and practices of patients and their families were reviewed. The perceptions and reactions of different staff members to such beliefs and practices were considered in relation to health care in the community. Professional attitudes and value judgments about the beliefs and behavior of others were discussed at frequent staff meetings. Thus, the functions of doctors, nurses, and community health educators were seen to begin with trying to understand the health practices of the various ethnic groups in the community, and how these practices reflect their culture. This was done so that the staff would come to recognize that many of these practices have meaning and value for the people, a fact not generally appreciated by professional groups in Western society. This led to an approach in practice that tried not to challenge existing beliefs and practices in the community, but rather to develop a social climate in which there was easy interaction between health center staff and members of the community.

While the setting was in many ways a difficult one in which to begin a reorientation process, it offered certain opportunities, which we used. The majority of people were recent immigrants from many different parts of the world, with widely varied ideas about health and differing health-relevant practices. Some had deep-rooted traditions and beliefs that were far removed from the concepts of modern medicine. This situation presented the kind of contrast to Western beliefs and practices that led to a ready appreciation of the importance to health of social and cultural factors. Thus, a new orientation to community health care was developed, differing in several important respects from the usual organization and health practices in the country. These in-service discussions became the key to exploring the roles of different team members and modifying previous positions with special reference to daily functioning with members of the community.

For some of the staff with a Western medical or nursing training, this was a difficult learning experience. Not only were the social and cultural components of health care absent from their foundation training, but care of patients outside of institutions and concepts of family and community health were new. This is still generally true for new recruits to the health team. Doctors and nurses do not yet have the kind of experience and basic training suitable for community-oriented primary health care. Thus, we continue with the task of retraining and reorientation of each physician and nurse who joins this health center.

THE HEALTH CENTER AS A FIELD TRAINING AREA

Since its inception over 25 years ago, the health center at Kiryat Yovel has been used to provide field experience in community health care.

Different kinds of students receive training at the health center, including graduate students in public health and community medicine, undergraduate medical and nursing students, and others. In addition, the practice of the health center is recognized as an institution within which physicians can specialize in public health, and a number have done so. During the past decade, this function of training has grown considerably, and today the health center has difficulty in meeting the demands made upon it for teaching. We have therefore extended our field training to include other areas for teaching by the department of social medicine of the medical school. We are now exploring ways of developing community health care in the northeast areas of Jerusalem with clinical departments of the Hadassah hospital on Mount Scopus, Jerusalem. We are also associated with the Ashkelon medical center, which is both a general hospital and a district health office of the Ministry of Health.

The development of field training areas as distinct from hospital teaching centers has become a subject of much interest and, more recently, is being actively sponsored by the World Health Organization.[15,16] A recent international discussion on this subject was the WHO Eastern Mediterranean regional seminar on development of field training areas held in 1975. It is therefore appropriate to review the role of our departmental health center as a field training area (FTA).

The Objectives of the Health Center as a Teaching Unit

During recent years, a considerable number of students have passed through the health center, some 200 or more per year. The amount of time and depth of study has varied from several weeks to full-time block periods of study over several months. The teaching objectives of the health center and of the kind of experience it provides for different students are:

To provide learning experiences in community health care and to develop suitable teaching methods for this purpose. These include observations, active participation, and practical exercises in the community-oriented primary health care of the health center, with varying emphasis on:

Community health programs in primary health care.

Combining promotive, preventive, and curative functions in a family practice.

Maternal and child health care.

Family diagnosis and family health care.

Epidemiologic and biostatistical exercises of direct relevance to the population served by the center, for purposes of community diagnosis, health surveillance, and evaluation of programs.

Growth and development, exercises on assessment of trends in individual children and in the population of infants and children.

Knowledge, attitudes, and practices (KAP). Health-relevant KAP studies in the community.

Students' Clerkships and Workshops at the Health Center

In providing learning experiences, a number of teaching programs have been developed within the practices of the center. As indicated previously, a major thrust is the development of community medicine programs in the framework of primary health care. This aspect of the health center's activity is the central feature of a 10-week workshop in the Master of Public Health curriculum of studies.

In addition, undergraduate medical and nursing students have the opportunity to observe the different primary health care practices. Many of these students play an active role in the comprehensive family practice, the maternal and child health clinics, or the home care program for housebound patients. In some cases, too, they carry out family or community studies within the framework of their clerkship.

During recent years the various student groups have included:

Master of Public Health (MPH) Students. There are now 45 to 50 graduate students each year, consisting of two classes, the one Israeli and the other international, coming from a number of different countries. There are more or less the same number of students in each class, and both are composed of graduates of different disciplines: physicians, dentists, nurses, social scientists, social workers, environmental scientists, statisticians, nutritionists.

They attend the health center for a field seminar/workshop on community-oriented primary health care.[17,18] This workshop was first introduced in 1971 as an important part of the Master of Public Health curriculum. Its main objective is to study community medicine programs in the primary health care services of the health center. The unique aspect of the workshop is observation on how epidemiologic and clinical skills are used in bringing together community medicine and primary health care. This involves observations and meetings with doctors and nurses in primary health care, as well as epidemiologists, statisticians, psychologists, nutritionists, and others.

Another important function of the health center for these graduate students is the provision of a suitable facility for them to carry out community health studies for their dissertations. A considerable proportion of these are studies in Kiryat Yovel relevant to the community health programs.

Undergraduate Medical Students.   Elective clerkships in community-oriented primary health care.

All the undergraduate clerkships in community medicine and primary health care at the health center are elected. The clerkship varies from 1 to 6 months. The students are from Israel and other countries. The Israeli students come from all four medical schools in the country, and those from abroad are mainly from the United States. There are at least 20 such students in clerkships each year at the center, but this total may be as much as 40 or more when a special group clerkship is arranged with a particular medical school.

The health center also has students from other departments of the medical school. These have included students in psychiatry and pediatrics, who attend sessions in the family practice and maternal and child health units.

Nursing Students.   Students from the School of Nursing at the Hadassah-University Medical Center come to the health center for experience in family and community health as part of the curriculum of training. This association of the nursing school with the health center goes back more than 25 years. The student groups now include those studying for the Hebrew University baccalaureate degree in nursing, the 3-year course for state-registered nurses (SRN), students of midwifery, and SRN nurses specializing in public health. In all, there are some 100 students who complete practical studies in family and community nursing at the health center each year.

The clerkships for the SRN students extend over the 3 years of their training, with attachment to tutor-nurses at the health center, observations, and participation in various practices, home and school visiting, and seminars. The program includes a course in family dynamics, which extends through the first year, some 50 students spending a day a week at the health center for study of families in the community; and approximately 20 students have block periods of 2 months in either the second or third year of study when they are affiliated to the family practice, maternal and child health services of the health center, and have experience in care of the chronically sick at home.

The baccalaureate student nurses have two field block periods of one trimester each (approximately 11 weeks), in the second and fourth years of study, in special community nursing. One-fourth of the class, ten in each of the classes, are assigned to Kiryat Yovel. The fourth-year students undertake a problem-oriented study of a population group, such as attitudes of sixth-grade schoolchildren to cigarette smoking, associated with the planning of an intervention program which the group initiated. It is planned to carry this on as part of the school program. The second-year student group are concerned with study of well individuals and families, using a special guide on family assessment.

Student midwives attending the course at the Hadassah nursing school spend a week at the health center in the maternal and child health unit. Each student is assigned a pregnant mother attending the health center, preferably as early as possible in her first pregnancy. She visits the mother at home, and the contact is then continued with follow-up visits until delivery in hospital, where the student midwife is present.

Nurses studying for the Public Health Nursing Diploma course in Jerusalem or elsewhere in the country usually come to the center for observation visits.

Methods of Teaching

The second major objective of our health center as a field training area has been to develop suitable situations for learning about the various skills for community health care. This involves providing the kind of experience in community health care suited to the needs of different groups of students.

Observation and participation are the essence of practical experience in health care, as evidenced by clinical bedside experience and practical laboratory work. Bearing this in mind, we have carefully defined what elements of our health center's practice should be used to provide students with a useful and satisfying learning experience. Thus, if students are to learn about community diagnosis, they must see it being carried out and, if possible, do it themselves. If they are to appreciate the potential of primary health care as an instrument of public health and community medicine, they need to be exposed to a practice which is doing this. They should also have the opportunity to critically analyze the way community medicine programs are developed in different forms of primary health care.

In order to achieve the above goals, we have organized student experience along the lines already described, but which merit further consideration:

1. A field workshop on community health care for graduate MPH students. The arrangement of the workshop ensures a program of observations of ways epidemiology and community medicine are integrated in different forms of primary health care, namely, the family practice, maternal and child health services, and home care of homebound patients by the health center. The observations are supplemented by reading and special statistical exercises. Their final presentations include critical analysis of community-oriented primary health care and its applicability in other situations.

2. Clinical clerkships and problem-oriented studies. Every effort is made to ensure that medical and nursing students are attached to staff members while carrying out the routines of their practice, such as interviewing and examining patients at the health center's clinics, home visits to mothers who have recently returned home from the hospital with their newborn babies, acutely ill patients who have asked for a doctor or nurse to visit, and chronically ill homebound patients. In addition, the medical and nursing students are exposed to different community medicine programs in the health center's practice.

   Students who carry out their clerkship at the health center for a month or more are usually assigned a problem-oriented task. Thus, one senior medical student carried out a study of our program for the control of hypertension, atherosclerosis, and diabetes (CHAD). Her task was an evaluative study of the modification of blood pressure and smoking behavior in this community medicine program.

3. The practices of the health center and the community it serves constitute a very useful framework for students, especially those studying for their Master of Public Health, to carry out special studies on the basis of which they submit their theses. Each year, staff of the department of social medicine and other departments list a number of subjects on which they are working; these include topics of interest to the health center's practice, and students may

elect from this list. Some 30 percent of dissertations during the past 10 years have been on studies of different aspects of the community health care practices of the health center.

Team for the Field Training Area

As in other training programs, the most important ingredient for success in developing an FTA for community-oriented primary health care is an adequate teaching health team.

Physicians on the health center staff are all registered as specialists in public health. This is a requirement of the medical school's department of social medicine, of which the health center is an integral part. In addition, the department and health center have several special posts for physicians who wish to specialize in public health. This includes facilities for those interested in community-oriented primary health care. There are aspects of this approach that are universally relevant, being especially applicable to countries that offer special postgraduate training in family medicine or general practice. Such training could, and we believe should, include experience in the skills needed for community-oriented primary health care. However, to do this it is essential that they have suitable field training areas (FTA). At present, schools of public health in leading Western countries do not take responsibility for the development of community medicine combined with primary health care.

Our 5-year specialization period for physicians includes:

1 . *Experience in Community-Oriented Primary Health Care at the Department's Community Health Center in Jerusalem.* This involves both clinical and community medicine, the latter requiring participation in several community medicine programs and responsibility for at least one. They also take an active part in the weekly community medicine rounds of the department and health center.

2. *Completion of Requirements for the Master's in Public Health (MPH) of the Hebrew University.* One of the areas to which special attention is given is community health care. The courses include community health sciences, such as epidemiology, biostatistics, and behavioral sciences, and their application in community health care. For this purpose, the obligatory field workshop is conducted, which involves the students in observations and exercises on the practices of the health center, especially the ways in which community medicine and primary health care have been developed as a unified practice in a neighborhood. Study of medical care in other settings provides the opportunity to consider and

prepare proposals for ways such a unified practice could be developed. It should be stressed here that this field workshop is not confined to physicians specializing in the department, but is required of MPH students of various disciplines. It is a valuable experience for physicians and others to share their observations, and preparation for group presentations with students of other professions, such as nursing, social work, statistics, health education.

3. *Other Requirements.* These include hospital medicine, of which internal medicine is obligatory, and an elective, which may be in a hospital laboratory of biochemistry or microbiology.

Nurses of the department, with university degrees, are encouraged to take the MPH course, majoring in community nursing. Their experience is similar to that of physicians on the MPH course. However, the majority of nurses on the health center staff are state registered nurses (SRN) without a university degree. They are required to obtain the Israel diploma in public health nursing, as well as having supervised experience with various teams of the health center. Their in-service training continues as participant members of the weekly community medicine rounds and in special sessions such as epidemiology and family psychiatry.

We have made a substantial investment in training of physicians, nurses, and other health professionals, with considerable success. A number are already working in related fields in various parts of this and other countries. However, there are still too few physicians who are attracted to this area of work, a reflection on the status of community health care and of medical training for it.[19] It is now clear that new approaches in medical education cannot always emerge from the old. More than minor modifications of basic curricula of training are needed. To the question as to whether traditional schools of medicine and nursing provide this training, the answer is: No. Hospital-based training of medical and nursing students is an unsuitable foundation for future community health practitioners. New approaches need new forms. New kinds of institutions, such as the health center at Kiryat Yovel, need new types of personnel.

REFERENCES

1. Merton RK: Social Theory and Social Structure. New York, Free Press, 1949.
2. Shuval JT, Antonovsky A, Davies AM: Social Functions of Medical Practice. San Francisco, Jossey-Bass, 1970.

3. Bott E: Family and Social Network, 2nd ed. London, Tavistock, 1971.
4. Mitchell JC (ed): Social Networks in Urban Situations. Manchester, Univ. of Manchester Press, 1969.
5. Wellman B: The community question: The intimate networks of East Yorkers. Am J Sociol 84:1201, 1979.
6. Mann KJ, Medalie JH, Lieber E, et al.: Visits to Doctors. Jerusalem, Jerusalem Academic Press, 1970.
7. Kark SL: Epidemiology and Community Medicine. New York, Appleton, 1974.
8. Abramson JH, Kark SL, Epstein LM, et al.: Community health study in Jerusalem: aims, design, response. Isr J Med Sci 15:725, 1979.
9 Kark SL, Gofin J, Abramson JH, et al.: The prevalence of selected health characteristics of men. A community health survey in Jerusalem. Isr J Med Sci 15:732, 1979.
10. Epstein FH, Napier JA, Block WD, et al.: The Tecumseh study: design, progress and perspectives. Arch Environ Health 21:402, 1970.
11. Pickles WN: Epidemiology in Country Practice. Bristol, John Wright, 1939.
12. Kark SL: Infections in a family practice. In Epidemiology and Community Medicine. New York, Appleton, 1974, p 361.
13. ———: Rheumatic fever and rheumatic heart disease community program. In Ibid, p 370.
14. ———: Anemia in pregnancy. In Ibid, p 395.
15. WHO: Report of a WHO Regional Seminar on Development of Field Training Areas, Isfahan, Iran, May 1975. WHO Regional Office for the Eastern Mediterranean.
16. Fisek NH: Away from the ivory tower: student health workers live and learn in field training areas. WHO Chron 31:175, 1977 (summary).
17. Kark SL, Mainemer N, Abramson JH, Levav I, Kurtzman C: Community medicine and primary health care: a field workshop on the use of epidemiology in practice. Int J Epidemiol 2:419, 1973.
18. Kark SL: Graduate Education in Public Health and Community Medicine—Hebrew University-Hadassah Medical School, 1960–1977. Department of Social Medicine, 1977.
19. Shuval J: Israel Study of Socialization for Medicine. National Center for Health Services Research. Research Digest Series. DHEW Publication (PHS) 79-3231, 1978.

CHAPTER 5

MOTHER AND CHILD
IN PRIMARY HEALTH CARE

Focus on the family is often featured as an important function of primary care practitioners. Organized health care of mothers and children is possibly the outstanding example of attention to central functions of the family, namely, family formation and early child rearing. In Israel, with its small population of some 3.5 million, there are approximately 800 maternal and child centers distributed through the country. They are essentially preventive and promotive services, staffed by specially trained public health nurses and conducted separately from the general curative clinic services of the country. The association of physicians with these centers varies. In many, the doctors are full-time staff members of the mother and child service and have an active role in direction and management of the centers, in addition to their clinical functions. In others, their functions are essentially clinical, visiting the center and examining mothers or babies referred by the nurses on the basis of agreed routines.

There is a tendency to use the terms *preventive medicine* and *community medicine* interchangeably, or even synonymously. This may lead to assumptions that certain things are being done, that, in fact, are not. In the present context, a distinction is drawn between community medicine and preventive medicine. A personal physician, generalist, family physician, pediatrician, or obstetrician may conduct a preventive service for an individual mother and her child without necessarily being community-oriented or involved in the practice of community medicine. It is the acceptance of responsibility for the health of a population, or the community's health as such, that distinguishes community medicine. In this particular case, it is the responsibility for the maternal and child health of the community that requires the use of community medicine skills, such as epidemiology, in health appraisal of maternal and child health. This involves community diagnosis, ongoing surveillance of the health of these important sections of the community and of the factors affecting their health. Such epidemiologic activities are seldom a feature of preventive maternal and child care.

The departmental health center in Kiryat Yovel provides two types of service to different parts of the area. The one is essentially a promotive and preventive service to mothers and children, similar to those in the rest of the country; the other is integrated within a family medicine practice, which combines curative, preventive, and promotive services. We have combined community medicine programs with the primary health care in both types of service. The community programs that will be reviewed in this and the following chapter relate to pregnancy and its outcome, and to the growth and development of infants and young children.

PREGNANCY AND ITS OUTCOME

In Israel, it is customary for women to have their babies in obstetric departments of hospitals. In 1977, 100 percent of Jewish births and 97 percent of Arab and other non-Jewish births took place in hospitals.[1] Whereas the figure for the Jewish population has been close to 100 percent since the origin of the state, the percentage of Arab births that take place in hospitals has increased considerably, from 55 percent in 1960 to the latest figure.

Prenatal care is provided at maternal and child health centers distributed throughout the country. There are many women who, in addition, use the services of obstetricians at hospitals or even in private practice, and this may represent a growing trend in the country. However, the number of pregnant women under supervision of the preventive maternal and child health centers continues to grow, from 16,521 in 1950 to 76,563 in 1975.[1]

Postnatal care during the first month of life is shared between the hospitals and preventive child health centers. The immediate post-delivery care takes place in hospitals, and this is followed by care from the maternal and child health center at home or at the center. Thus, any intensive care needed is done in hospitals, some of which are now specially equipped for intensive care of the kind needed for babies of very low birth weight, markedly low gestational age, or other problems.

There has been a marked decline in early neonatal mortality in a number of more developed countries during the recent past. Thus, in Sweden, Holland, and the United Kingdom, the change in first-week mortality rates was as follows:[2]

	1964	1974
Sweden	10.5	5.5 (1975)
Holland	10.1	6.6
England and Wales	12.0	9.4

A similar decline has been recorded in Israel, where the corresponding figures for 1955, 1965, 1975, and 1977 for the Jewish population were 11.4, 13.0, 10.1, and 8.0. In the United States, there was a decline in early neonatal mortality rates, which was part of a long-term trend in reduction of mortality of babies weighing over 2500 gm at birth. By contrast, the mortality rate of low birth weight (LBW) babies, that is, those weighing 2500 gm and under, changed little over the period 1950 to 1965, but decreased steeply by 1974.[3] The probable causes for this recent change are advances in medical technology, such as electronic fetal monitoring, and the spread of intensive neonatal care units.

Maternal mortality rates, as well as perinatal and neonatal mortality rates, have declined in all sections of the Israeli population.[1,4] The maternal mortality per 1000 live births in 1977 was 0.1 (ten deaths) in the Jewish population, and 0.3 (6 deaths) in the Arab and other non-Jewish sectors. The decline in the former was eightfold— from 0.8 in the period 1950 to 1954 to 0.1 in 1977.

Neonatal mortality rates in the Jewish population have declined from 22.7 per 1000 live births in 1950 to 9.8 in 1977. Over this period of time, there has also been a marked reduction in mortality rates in the week following birth, from 14.3 to 8.0 first-week mortality rate, as well as in the last 3 weeks of the neonatal period, from 8.4 to 1.8 per 1000 live births. The main room for improvement is thus in the perinatal period, late fetal (28th week gestation) and first week after birth. In 1977, the perinatal mortality rate was 23.2 for the Arab and other non-Jewish population and 15.9 for Jews.

Among the factors determining these favorable trends for the country as a whole are probably improvement in the standard of living, health of the mothers, and family spacing.

Fertility rates have on the one hand been shown to be related to social and economic conditions and, on the other, to influence outcome of pregnancy. High fertility rates are found in deprived, less-educated populations, and are associated with poorer outcome of pregnancy.[5]

TABLE 5-1

The Change in Specific Birth Rates in Different Population Groups of Israel, According to Mother's Age*

POPULATION GROUP	AGE IN YEARS						
	19 and under	20-24	25-29	30-34	35-39	40-44	45 and over
Jewish							
1955	60.9	228.6	198.9	140.3	74.0	21.5	4.6
1975	34.0	186.4	198.4	140.1	66.9	14.1	1.0
Christian							
1955	64.3	239.0	262.6	248.9	117.6	30.7	(6.0)
1975	37.3	198.3	199.5	139.2	76.7	17.3	(2.1)
Moslem							
1955	139.1	357.2	357.6	356.7	222.1	120.8	37.9
1975	104.8	345.5	383.3	348.4	242.8	96.1	28.6

*Births per 1000 women.

Fertility rates have changed considerably in the Jewish and Christian populations (Table 5-1). The decline in specific birth rates, according to mother's age, in the Jewish population is especially to be noted in the young, 19 or less, and the older groups, 40 to 44 and 45 and over. In the Christian population, it is evidenced in all age groups. The Jewish groups in which the decline has been most notable are those whose origins are in North Africa and Asia. Their total fertility* has declined from 5.68 in 1955 to 3.42 in 1977, in contrast to those of European/American origin, 2.63 to 2.83, and Israeli-born women, 2.83 to 2.89; the overall total fertility of the Jewish population declined from 3.64 to 2.99. There has been a marked decline in total fertility of the small Christian population of the country, the comparable figures being 4.85 to 3.14, but that of the larger Moslem population has remained high, 7.96 and 7.29.

Perhaps the most sensitive indicator of social change affecting the fertility rate is the standard of education of women. There has been a continuing change in the standard of education of Jewish women, as indicated by the data for all women over the age of 14, and especially for women aged 18 to 34 years, which includes the age groups with the highest fertility rates.

*Total fertility is the estimate of the average number of children a woman may bear during her lifetime, on the basis of the specific age fertility rates for that year.[1]

The change in the standard of education of Jewish women in the country, aged 14 years and over, is shown by the following data:

Years of Education	Percentage of Women	
	1966	*1977*
4 or less	25	14
5–8	31	24
9–12 (high school)	34	44
13 and over (be- yond high school)	10	18

The data for this comparison were obtained from the *Statistical Abstracts of Israel* published in 1967 and 1978.

Another possibly important influence on the favorable trend of pregnancy outcome has been the change in physique of women. The outcome of pregnancy has been shown to be associated with height of the mother, perinatal mortality being lower in taller than in shorter women.[6,7] With improvements in the standard of living, especially in diet, the nutritional state and growth must have been favorably influenced. A reflection of this is probably demonstrated in the differences in height of older and younger women and men found in a total community health study[8,9] of Kiryat Yovel, Jerusalem, carried out between 1969 and 1971:

Age Group	Women		Men	
	Mean	*S.D*	*Mean*	*S.D.*
15–24	159.5	5.9	171.4	6.9
25–34	158.3	6.2	171.4	7.3
35–44	156.1	6.0	168.4	6.4
45–54	154.4	5.9	166.5	6.6
55–64	152.1	6.5	164.9	6.2

Thus, present trends in lower perinatal morbidity and mortality are probably a result of the life experience of women, with improved nutrition and growth through childhood producing adults whose physique may be associated with better reproductive performance.

These advances in the standard of education and increase in height of women are not isolated phenomena. They have occurred over the same period as changes in social and economic conditions have taken place. Among the more important of these is that of food availability as shown in the food balance sheet, published annually since the establishment of the state.[1] The outstanding feature of relevance to our present consideration is the increase of protein from animal sources, especially meat, as is shown by the following data:

	Protein Grams per Capita per Day	
	1949/1950	*1976/1977*
From animal foods	32	50
Meat	7	25
Milk and milk products	13	17
Eggs	5	6
Fish	7	2
Total	84	97

THE 28TH-DAY REVIEW: PROGRESS THROUGH PREGNANCY AND ITS OUTCOME

A service focused on pregnancy and its outcome is a feature of the Kiryat Yovel health center. The 28th-day review is a report on surveillance of health and health care through pregnancy to approximately 1 month after birth. Associated with health surveillance, specific community medicine programs are developed. As in the rest of Jerusalem and the country, it is customary for Kiryat Yovel women to be delivered in obstetric departments of hospitals in the city.

The Health Team.   The various members of the health team are concerned with this program as part of their wider functions in maternal and child care and family practice. The central members of the team are family physicians and nurses, as well as pediatricians. The chief nurse of the program is a trained midwife in addition to her other nursing qualifications. The team has been trained for both the clinical and public health aspects of the program. It is supported by a visiting obstetrician-gynecologist, who conducts pre- and postnatal examinations and acts as a consultant to the physicians of the team.

Special records are used and are maintained by the health records section of the health center. The information accumulated in the course of this surveillance program is reviewed periodically. Thus, during the 7-year period 1971 to 1977, there were 2536 births, of which 2512 were live births, in the defined geographic area of the health center practice. The mortality rates in this population were:

Stillbirths	9.5	(per 1000 total births)
Perinatal mortality	21.0	
First day mortality	8.3	
First week mortality	11.5	(per 1000 live births)
Neonatal mortality	14.3	
Postneonatal mortality	3.1	
Total infant mortality (IMR)	17.5	

The individual mother and baby records include the mother's progress through pregnancy, delivery, and puerperium; and the baby at birth, progress through the neonatal period, and status at the 28th-day examination. The findings are reviewed and related to the ongoing community health programs, such as the control of anemia in pregnancy and asymptomatic bacteriuria, as well as the need for new programs, for example, family planning, and the prevention of cigarette smoking.

In a typical year, 1976, the occurrence of major abnormalities in 310 births in the health center's community was as follows:

Pregnancy. Major abnormalities: 6.6 percent, the majority being cases of bleeding (4.3 percent). Of interest is that there were only two women in the practice who had anemia of below 10 gm hemoglobin/100 ml during their pregnancy in this year. In the early years of the practice, anemia in pregnancy was common, for which a special community program was started in 1963 and continued to the present time.[10]

Delivery. Major abnormalities: 17 percent, including Caesarian deliveries, postpartum hemorrhage, and malpresentations.

Babies at Birth. Major abnormalities: 11 percent, the majority (6 percent) being of birth weight 2250 gm and below. The weight distribution of these 19 babies was:

Grams	Number
1000 or less	1 (neonatal death)
1001–1500	3 (1 stillbirth)
1501–2000	8 (1 neonatal death)
2001–2250	7 (1 stillbirth)

In addition, there were ten babies of birth weight between 2251 and 2500 gm, making a total of 9.4 percent low birth weight babies (LBW). A special part of the community program for promotion of growth and development (PROD) focuses on the LBW babies.

Neonatal Babies. (First 28 Days): Eight percent had severe conditions. Of these 25 babies, ten had acute infectious illness, respiratory and/or gastrointestinal, and there were three neonatal deaths.

At the 28-Day Examination: Five percent had notable abnormalities, the commonest being a diagnosis of marked underweight.

In the light of improving social and economic conditions, the widespread distribution of maternal and child health centers, the 100 percent hospital deliveries, and the favorable trend in outcome of pregnancy in this country, we need to ask several questions:

Is there a particular contribution to be made by community-oriented primary health care to further improve health through pregnancy and the neonatal period? And, more specifically: Is there a case for continuing the type of surveillance that has been described above?

The answer to these questions is in the affirmative. Surveillance, together with special studies, has pointed up several important problems to which primary health care can make a significant contribution. These have included:

Anemia in pregnancy.
Asymptomatic bacteriuria.
Cigarette smoking.
Initiation of breast feeding.
Family spacing.

For the first two of these, community programs have been in progress for many years. Cigarette smoking is a relatively recent problem in this population, and a program has now been initiated. More recently, information on the initiation of breast feeding and its maintenance has indicated the need for a special additional program emphasizing its importance. A family spacing program is now established and is about to be extended by the health center's team to several other communities. Previous reference has been made to this program in Chapter 4. Each of these various programs are reviewed at the community medicine rounds, which have been outlined in the same chapter. Two of these, namely, anemia in pregnancy and cigarette smoking by pregnant women, will now be discussed further.

ANEMIA IN PREGNANCY: THE CASE FOR ACTION AND THE INTERVENTION PROGRAM

When we initiated this community program at the health center in 1961, anemia in pregnancy was recognized as a prevalent condition in Jerusalem, as well as in other parts of Israel.[11,12]

Community Diagnosis

The reported findings of a relatively high prevalence of mild anemia in pregnancy was the reason for further epidemiologic investigation of the distribution of anemia and mean hemoglobin levels in Jerusalem as a whole, and in Kiryat Yovel itself. These studies, carried out in the early 1960s, were reported on in some detail.[10,13] A summary of the relevant findings in Jerusalem women are presented here. The prevalence of anemia cases with a hemoglobin level of below 10 gm/100 ml in 1961 and 1962 was:

	Percent
Prenatal second trimester	8.1
Prenatal third trimester	12.3
Following birth	16.7

Anemia was more common in higher parities, and in immigrants from Asian and North African countries, than in women born in Israel, in lower social classes, according to occupational rating of their husbands and a rating scale of neighborhood of residence.

Diet in Relation to the Hemoglobin Picture. Since it was found that social class and the neighborhood where people lived were associated with levels of hemoglobin, a dietary study was carried out to assess the possible effects of diet on hemoglobin levels of pregnant women living in a middle-class neighborhood and in a poorer neighborhood. In the middle-class neighborhoods, no differences in the diet were found between women with a hemoglobin level below or above 12 gm/100 ml, whereas in the poorer neighborhood the differences were marked, the women with Hb below 12 gm/100 ml had markedly inferior diets compared with those Hb levels above 12 gm/100 ml.

The Neighborhood Anemia Program

The pregnant women of Kiryat Yovel compared favorably with the rest of Jerusalem. Controlling for social class and neighborhood rating, the mean hemoglobin level was higher than expected, and the anemia rate consequently lower than in the rest of Jerusalem. The main difference at that time between the women of this area and the rest of Jerusalem was the more intensive routine prenatal investigation, which included hemoglobin determinations and treatment. It was therefore decided to develop this care further in a more defined community program.

The intervention program commenced in 1963 and continues in modified form to the present time. It has two objectives: continuing epidemiologic surveillance of the hemoglobin level with the aim of shifting the distribution curve to the right, and reduction of the incidence of anemia in pregnant women.

Hemoglobin Investigations.   Using standardized methods of investigation, hemoglobin estimates are made during the second and third trimesters. When the program began, the aim was to carry out additional determinations in the first trimester and 6 weeks after delivery, and the hospitals in which the women delivered carried out this investigation on the first postnatal day.

We stopped the routine 6-weeks Hb postnatal examination, because the levels were satisfactory at this time in all women who had adequate levels through their pregnancy. We therefore confined this extra investigation to those women who had had anemia during pregnancy.

The treatment during pregnancy has remained consistent since the commencement of the program:

Hemoglobin Level (per 100 ml)	*Treatment*
12 gm and over	No treatment
11 gm	1 iron tablet daily
10 gm	3 iron tablets daily
Less than 10 gm	Hematocrit and full blood count Treatment according to the nature of the anemia

The iron tablets used have been ferrous gluconate (0.3 gm), ferrous sulphate (0.2 gm), or ferrocal (0.5 gm).

The initial team consisted of an epidemiologist, two physicians of the maternal and child health unit of the health center, and the coordinating nurse of this unit. In the early phase of this community program, the team met weekly to review each aspect of the program, especially:

Blood examinations: Standardizing procedures in the taking of blood and in the examinations, checking the extent to which the examinations were carried out at the prescribed times.

Treatment: Checking compliance with treatment prescribed, and ensuring that it is prescribed according to the agreed schedule.

Analysis of the data: Changes in the distribution of hemoglobin levels and the incidence of anemia.

The program is now a well-established part of the maternal and child health service; the rate of anemia is low and has been so for many years. The change is shown in the following data:

Period	Hemoglobin Below 10 gm/ml at Any Time During Pregnancy (% of Pregnant Women)
1958–1959	12.0
1964–1966	8.8
1970–1971	3.3
1975–1976	1.6

At more or less the same time as this program was introduced into the health center at Kiryat Yovel, a similar but less intensively monitored program was initiated throughout all the mother and child centers of the city of Jerusalem. This followed several preparatory seminars and discussions on the epidemiology of anemia in pregnancy in this area. The early experience was reported, noting the increase in the hemoglobin level and the decline in anemia rate in Jerusalem.

With the considerable decline in anemia and the increase in level of hemoglobin that has taken place, the question arises as to whether we need to continue with the program of surveillance as we have done since the inception of the project. In the light of the present inflationary economic situation in the country, with food and other living costs increasing considerably, surveillance of this aspect of the community's health is continuing.

CIGARETTE SMOKING
IN PREGNANCY

The Need for Preventive Action

The case for action to stop cigarette smoking by women during pregnancy is now well established.[14] Women who smoke cigarettes during pregnancy have a higher proportion of low birth weight babies than women who do not smoke.

There are now many studies which confirm the first report by Simpson, in 1957, that babies born to mothers who smoke during pregnancy are on average lower in weight than those born to nonsmokers.[14-18] In addition, perinatal and neonatal mortality rates have been found to be associated with smoking during pregnancy.[16,17] Higher spontaneous abortion rates have also been reported[19,20] and there is some suggestive evidence that smoking increases the occurrence of congenital abnormalities.[20,21]

In the Kiryat Yovel community, there has been an increase in the proportion of women who smoke cigarettes during pregnancy. Over 80 percent of all pregnant women eligible to use the health center for care through pregnancy use it. Of the women who attended the prenatal clinics of the health center between 1970 and 1972, 17 percent said they were smokers. This proportion of smokers increased to 27 percent in 1975 and 1976.[22] The increase reflected in this comparatively short period of time may be regarded as part of a process of social change, more especially in the new generation of young women, who are daughters of immigrants from North African and Asian countries. Their traditional mothers were usually not cigarette smokers, whereas they, the daughters, have become so, probably in the process of their acculturation to the society, and possibly as a manifestation of their liberation.

Health education in pregnancy includes the subject of cigarette smoking, and every opportunity is taken to explain the hazards of smoking. Doctors and most nurses do not smoke, and even those who do smoke, refrain from doing so in the clinic. It is recognized that this is a difficult task; the habit begins many years before marriage and having a family, and continues afterward. There is, therefore, need to link this program during pregnancy with one focusing on schoolchildren, adolescents, and army recruits.

Epidemiologic studies of cigarette smoking by schoolchildren point to a number of factors, including smoking by parents, siblings, and peer groups; several studies have also shown an association between cigarette smoking and lower academic achievement at school.[23,24] The influence of the home has been well documented, suggesting that family health education in primary health care might make an important contribution to reduction of the incidence of new smokers through childhood to adolescence. The primary care program could include both the school health service and family discussions with parents in the course of family practice and community health nursing.

The evidence that exposure to cigarette smoking may cause harm to babies[25,26] indicates the importance of extending the program beyond pregnancy to the mother and father, and others who may have close contact with the baby.

The harmful effects of cigarette smoking as a risk factor for heart disease is discussed in Chapter 7, suggesting the need for a comprehensive and community-wide program for stopping cigarette smoking. Primary health care has an important contribution to make.

REFERENCES

1. Statistical Abstract of Israel 1978. No. 29. Jerusalem, Central Bureau of Statistics, 1978

2. World Health Organization: World Health Statistics Annual, Vol 1. Vital Statistics and Causes of Death. 1964, 1973–1976. Geneva, WHO, 1967, 1976

3. Kleinman JC, Kovar MG, Feldman JJ, Young CA: A comparison of 1960 and 1973–74 early neonatal mortality in selected states. Am J Epidemiol 108:454, 1978.

4. Zadka P: Infant Mortality 1975–77. Jerusalem, Central Bureau of Statistics, 1978

5. Omran AR, Standley CC (eds): Family Formation Patterns and Health. Geneva, WHO, 1976

6. Butler NR, Alberman ED (eds): Perinatal Problems. The Second Report of the 1958 British Perinatal Mortality Study. Edinburgh, Livingstone, 1969

7. ——, Bonham DG (eds): Perinatal Mortality. The First Report of the 1958 British Perinatal Mortality Study. Edinburgh, Livingstone, 1963

8. Abramson JH, Kark SL, Epstein LM, et al.: A community health study in Jerusalem: aims, design, response. Isr J Med Sci 15:725, 1979

9. Kark SL, Gofin J, Abramson JH, et al.: The prevalence of selected health characeristics of men. A community health survey in Jerusalem. Isr J Med Sci 15:732, 1979

10. ——: Anemia in pregnancy. In Kark SL: Epidemiology and Community Medicine. New York, Appleton, 1974, p 395

11. Avivi L, Ilan J, Guggenheim K: Hemoglobin levels in the Jewish rural population of Israel (in Hebrew). Briut Hatsibur 5:5, 1962

12. Rachmilewitz M, Izak G, Grossowicz N, et al.: Anemia in pregnancy. Harefuah 57:81, 1959

13. Kark SL, Peritz E, Shiloh A, et al.: Epidemiological analysis of the hemoglobin picture in parturient women of Jerusalem. Am J Public Health 54:947, 1964

14. Report of the Surgeon General USA: The Health Consequences of Smoking. DHEW 1039(10):123, 1977

15. Simpson WJ: A preliminary report of cigarette smoking and the incidence of prematurity. Am J Obstet Gynecol 3:808, 1957

16. Comstock GW, Shah FK, Meyer B, et al.: Low birthweight and neonatal mortality rate related to maternal smoking and socioeconomic status. Am J Obstet Gynecol 111:53, 1971

17. Butler NR, Goldstein H, Ross EM: Cigarette smoking in pregnancy: its influence on birthweight and perinatal mortality. Br Med J 2:127, 1972

18. Goldstein H: Smoking in pregnancy: some notes on the statistical controversy. Br J Prev Soc Med 31:13, 1977

19. Kline J, Stein ZA, Susser M et al.: Smoking: a risk factor for spontaneous abortion. N Engl J Med 297:793, 1977

20. Himmelberger DU, Byron WB, Cohen EN: Cigarette smoking during pregnancy and the occurrence of spontaneous abortion and congenital abnormality. Am J Epidemiol 108:470, 1978

21. Frederick J, Alberman E, Goldstein H. Possible teratogenic effect of cigarette smoking. Nature 231:529, 1971

22. Gofin J: Smoking in Pregnancy. A community survey. Harefuah, 96:278, 1979 (In Hebrew with English summary)

23. Bewley BR, Bland JM: Academic performance and social factors related to cigarette smoking by schoolchildren. Br J Prev Soc Med 31:18, 1977

24. Salber EJ, Freeman HE, Abelin T: Needed research on smoking: lessons from the Newton study. In Borgatta EF, Evans RR (eds): Smoking and Health Behaviour. Chicago, Aldine 1968

25. Harlap S, Davies AM: Infant admissions to hospital and maternal smoking. Lancet 1:529, 1974

26. Colley JRT, Holland WW, Corkhill RT: Childhood pneumonia and parental smoking. Lancet 2:1031, 1974

CHAPTER 6

GROWTH AND DEVELOPMENT OF INFANTS AND YOUNG CHILDREN

INTRODUCING A COMMUNITY ORIENTATION IN THE PRIMARY HEALTH CARE OF CHILDREN

Attention to growth and development is an integral part of the health care of children. All maternal and child health centers carry out some routines related to growth and development. The weighing of babies is a feature of such centers, and this is one of the main reasons mothers bring their babies to the centers. Usually the routine is to weigh the baby, record the weight, compare it with a recognized standard, and assess whether the baby's weight growth curve is satisfactory. Weighing is thus one aspect of the appraisal of an individual baby's health, which guides the doctor or nurse in the feeding or other advice given the mother. A similar process applies to other measurements that may be made.

However, appraisal of growth and development goes beyond this, and needs to include an epidemiologic orientation. This involves the widening of the functions of primary care, to include responsibility for the health and development of the population of babies and young children as a group. In this regard, several basic questions need to be answered. For the purposes of the community health center in Kiryat Yovel, we have postulated the following questions:

What is the state of health of the population of children in the community served by the center, and what are the factors determining it? Growth and development are important components of health and may be studied epidemiologically, as well as in the diagnostic workup

Dr. Hava Palti is co-author of this chapter.

of individual children. In doing this, community diagnosis of child health extends from mortality and morbidity rates to answering additional questions, such as:

Does the pattern of child growth and development in this community differ from that of other communities?

Are there differences between various groups of children within the community itself? This includes consideration of differences by ethnic group, family size, social class of the family, and parents' education.

Can inferences be made as to the factors determining these differences and can these factors be suitably modified? The critical question in this regard:

Can primary care itself make the contribution necessary to promote growth and development in the child population as a whole, and especially for the at-risk groups of children?

We have attempted to answer these questions by initiating a community program for the promotion of growth and development (PROD) in the family practice and mother and child services of the Kiryat Yovel health center. As a background to consideration of the case for a community-oriented program focused on growth and development in primary health care, it is of interest to review some of the changes in health indices of infants in the country. Kiryat Yovel is a Jewish neighborhood, hence this review will be centered on the infant health indices in the Jewish population of Israel. Advances in maternal health and social conditions have been associated with marked improvement in the outcome of pregnancy and a considerable decline in infant mortality (Table 6-1).

As expected, the decline in mortality was very marked from 1 to

TABLE 6-1

The Decline in Infant Mortality Rate* in Jewish Infants of Israel, 1950-1978[1]

AGE	1950	1955	1960	1965	1970	1975	1978
0–6 days	14.3	11.4	12.9	13.0	11.6	10.1	8.1
7–27 days	8.4	5.3	3.4	2.2	2.0	2.2	1.9
1–11 months	23.5	15.7	10.7	7.5	5.3	5.6	3.6
Total	46.2	32.4	27.0	22.7	18.9	17.9	13.6

*Per 1000 live births.

11 months, and in the last 3 weeks of the neonatal period. Indicative of the general social and economic advancement in the country are two measures of immediate relevance to infant morbidity and mortality. The crowding index, as measured by the number of persons per room, declined from a median of 2.2 in 1959 to 1.5 in 1976; the percentage of families with less than two persons per room increased from 4.3 to 8.3. The percentage of families having electric refrigerators in the home increased from 34 to 97 over a similar period.

THE CASE FOR A COMMUNITY PROGRAM TO PROMOTE GROWTH AND DEVELOPMENT (PROD)

With the favorable trend in the infant mortality rate (IMR) that was evident in the 1960s, we felt that more attention could be given to other aspects of child health, such as the promotion of growth and development. It could not be assumed that the decline in IMR was in itself an indication of favorable trends in growth and development of infants in all segments of the community. In fact, there was evidence of differences in the rates of growth and intellectual development between children of different subgroups of the population.

Our departmental studies of weight and height of infants and children in the Kiryat Yovel community had shown that babies of Israeli-born parents were heavier than those of Moroccan-born parents from the age of 8 weeks, although at that time the latter were heavier at birth.[2] We had also found that at the age of 3 years, children in poorer neighborhoods were shorter and lighter than those from a better-off part of Kiryat Yovel.[3] Anemia in infancy and in pregnancy were also found in the same neighborhood where there was growth retardation. These findings have been previously reported in some detail.[4]

The physical growth retardation in infancy and early childhood, which we have noted, occurred in other poorer immigrant communities in Israel, in which unsatisfactory intellectual development and educational achievement of the children had been reported by psychologists and educationalists.[5-7] A direct relation between social class and intelligence scores has been consistently reported in studies of children in different countries.[8-12]

An investigation of intellectual performance by children between the ages of 4 and 6 years had only recently been reported when we were planning this program.[5] By the use of a Hebrew version of the

Wechsler Preschool and Primary Scale for Intelligence (WPPSI), differences were found in the performance by children of different social class and ethnic origin; children of Israeli and Western origin scored higher than those of Middle East and North African origin.

The question that these findings raised for us was whether primary health care of the kind provided in maternal and child health centers could be modified to make a contribution to promoting behavior and intellectual development as well as physical growth.

Among the possible causes that lie behind these differences in growth and development between children of different social classes and ethnic groups are: education of the parents, size of family, nutrition, infectious diseases, birth spacing, and social stimulation. We decided to investigate these factors further in the population served in Kiryat Yovel and to test the feasibility of developing a suitable community program within the framework of primary care at the health center.

For these purposes it was decided to establish a special PROD team from among the staff of the department of social medicine and the community health center at Kiryat Yovel.

THE PROD HEALTH TEAM

The health team responsible for the direction and performance of the program in the primary care practices of the health center consists of:

1. Members with special skills in community health sciences: public health pediatrician and epidemiologist, as director; biostatistician.
2. Members of the central teams of the primary care practices concerned with child health at the health center: family physician; pediatricians; public health nurses with special training in child health.
3. Supportive members of the team: health records and laboratory staff of the health center.
4. Consultants: epidemiologist; pediatrician; educational psychologist.
5. Special additional staff: psychologist; nutritionist.
6. Graduate students: MPH students carrying out studies for purposes of their dissertations.

All the above members of the team are involved part-time in this program. The consultants were used frequently in the planning and initial phases of the program, but with increasing experience of the team the need for consultation has decreased.

The team proposed an approach to the development of a PROD program in primary health care, which would be a guide to subsequent more detailed planning and action. This involved:

Community Diagnosis and Surveillance of Growth and Development (GD) in Infancy and Early Childhood. These were associated with the study of the distribution in the community of factors adversely affecting GD.

Intervention. Where found to be necessary, intervention to be directed toward:

1. Promotion of health through improved nutrition, family spacing, protection against infection, and social stimulation, with emphasis on parent-child interaction, including verbal stimulation and play activity.
2. Prevention of retardation in GD by focus on infants of families at special risk.

Program Evaluation. This included the extent to which the different elements of the program are carried out by the team, the response of the community, and the evaluation of desirable changes in behavior and GD itself.

COMMUNITY DIAGNOSIS AND SURVEILLANCE OF GROWTH AND DEVELOPMENT

Community diagnosis of child growth and development in primary health care is a continuing process. It requires the response of the mothers in the community beyond that of routine maternal and child health care clinics. The mothers may still come to the clinic whenever they wish to do so, but they are also asked to attend at regular intervals as required by the PROD program. From the time mothers return home from the hospital, they and their babies are involved in this care program, the initiative coming from themselves or the health center's family nurse of their neighborhood. The continuing contact between mother and child with the primary health care team allows for longitudinal investigation of growth and development from birth. Appointments are made at fixed times for examination of physical growth and psychomotor development, which are coordinated with other activities, such as immunizations. This has been done with all mothers and babies registered for care in both the family practice and the preventive maternal and child service of the health center. Information on new births in the areas of Kiryat Yovel served by the health center is obtained from several sources, namely, the district health office of the Ministry of Health, which obtains a copy of the birth registration record, the hospital in which the baby was born, and the neighborhood family nurse. As it is only the very occasional mother who does not make use of the health center services for her baby, the program commences with almost 100 percent of the babies born in the area. But the mobile character of the young adult population influences the continuity of the program.

The well-child service of the health center is provided to three neighborhoods of Kiryat Yovel. Of special interest to our present considerations is the fact that the families of these neighborhoods differed considerably in their social class distribution, allowing for a classification of the neighborhoods as predominantly middle-class, poor, and very poor.

Methods

The following measurements of growth and development are carried out:

Physical growth: Weight, length, head circumference, arm circumference, and triceps skinfold thickness.
Behavioral development: Tests of postural, coordination, social, and language development, using the Brunet-Lezine test.[13]
Intelligence: As measured by the Hebrew version of the WPPSI test[5] and MILI Israeli intelligence test for young children.[14]

Conducted by nurses of the team, the physical growth measurements have been scheduled for ages 1, 3, 6, 9, and 12 months in the first year, and then at 18, 24, 30, 36, and 48 months. The behavioral development tests, which are carried out by physicians, have been conducted at 9 and 24 months of age, and the intelligence tests at 3 years (MILI) and 5 years (WPPSI). Standardization of the methods used for the measurements is important in all such investigations: This is particularly important in a program being conducted as a longitudinal study in the framework of ongoing health supervision by health center teams, which include several doctors and a number of nurses.

Similar careful attention has been given in obtaining information about various determinants of growth and development, which include:

Breast-feeding and dietary practices.
Rank of baby and position in the family.
Mother: Age, parity, education, occupation, ethnic origin.
Family: Social class, by grading of father's occupation; father's education, ethnic origin; family spacing.
Home: Number of persons, crowding index.

The aspects of community diagnosis and health surveillance to be detailed further here are physical growth and nutrition, hemoglobin distribution and prevalence of anemia, and psychomotor development.

Physical Growth, Nutrition, and Diet

As indicated, when we were considering the initiation of this program in the 1960s, we had evidence of important differences in the growth of different groups of children in the area. Disadvantaged children manifested increasing retardation in weight growth through infancy, and at 3 and 4 years of age they were shorter than those from better-off homes.[3,4] Promotion of physical growth was thus one of the major goals of the program and we aimed to investigate this further, first to find out whether the differences noted earlier were still manifest in later cohorts of children, and if so, to study the causes, such as diet and nutrition. The interest of the family nurses in the well-child services of the health center was readily obtained, and various procedures were agreed on and standardized. The procedures included body measurements, dietary histories, and taking of blood specimens for hemoglobin determinations.

Community diagnosis of physical growth of the children has involved:

Longitudinal study of different birth cohorts of children.
Comparison of findings with international standards.
Examining for differences between various social groups of children within the community.
Study of the relationships between infant and child growth and nutritional status and diet.

Height and Weight. Comparing the findings in Kiryat Yovel with those of internationally acceptable standards has provided interesting information for community diagnosis.[15,16] The physical growth of the children has been measured against the growth curves published by the National Center for Health Statistics.[17] The Kiryat Yovel children were shorter through the first 2 years at all ages at which they were measured, i.e., 1, 3, 6, 12, and 24 months. This was more marked in boys than in girls.

In contrast to the first 2 years, at 3 and 4 years of age the percentile distribution of height of these children differed very little from that of the United States reference population. The weight differences were less consistent. These children were lighter than the reference population at 1 month of age, heavier at 3 and 6 months, and much the same at 24 months. Their weight for length also differed from the reference group. At 1 month they were lighter for length, heavier at 3 months, and with increasing age the weight for length measurement was similar, except that at 2 years of age the girls of Kiryat Yovel were heavier for their height.

However, there was a higher proportion of low weight Kiryat Yovel children at 30 and 36 months; 14 and 16 percent, respectively, being in the 10th percentile of the reference population. This difference did not persist, and in fact the Kiryat Yovel children were slightly heavier for their height at 48 months.

Within the area itself, some differences were noted. There were no significant differences in the birth weight of the babies of the three neighborhoods, nor according to social class. However, at 12, 18, and 24 months, children of the very poor neighborhood were both lighter and shorter than those of the middle-class neighborhood. There was little difference in the weight : height ratio, except that more middle-class neighborhood 1-year-olds were overweight, and there was little evidence of malnutrition underweight in any group.

Diet. In addition to the routine history of feeding practices obtained by nurses from mothers at the time of their attendance, a special investigation was undertaken by a nutritionist. This involved detailed questioning of mothers of two cohorts of babies, one group from 6 months of age and the other from 18 months. Both groups were interviewed every 6 months to the age of 4 years. The nutritionist checked the diet of the baby with the mother for each hour of the day and night over the previous 24 hours. The mother estimated quantities according to household utensils. These estimates were then converted to metric measurements, and the nutritionist appraised the nutrient intake using a local food consumption table.

Comparison of nutrient intake with recommended dietary allowances (RDA) of the U.S.A. National Academy of Sciences[18] and the World Health Organization—Food and Agricultural Organization,[19] indicated that the Kiryat Yovel children had a very much higher protein intake than the RDA at each fixed time of interview from 6 months through to 4 years of age. The calorie intake was slightly lower than the RDA during the first 2 years. After this, the relative calorie intake declined with increasing age, the percentage of children below 100 percent RDA increasing from 60 at 18 months to 84 at 48 months. There was a considerably lower iron intake than the RDA by United States standards, but the intake was similar to that recommended by WHO. The source of iron changed with age; heme sources, such as liver and meat, contributed 48 percent of iron at 30 months but only 19 percent at 48 months, when the children were probably eating much the same foods as other members of the family.

Comparisons within the community itself indicated limited differences. Six-month-old babies of lower social classes had lower calorie intake than those of upper social classes; and babies of higher birth rank, three and over, had a lower calorie intake than those of birth ranks one and two. No other important differences were found in the diet of various groups of children. As the children attained the ages of 30, 36, and 48 months, no social class differences in nutrient intake were noted. Although both the protein and calorie intakes were higher in children of mothers of higher education, there was no marked inadequacy in the children of less-educated mothers.

Hemoglobin and Anemia. The examinations of all babies attending the health center at 9 months of age include a capillary blood sample taken by finger prick. Hemoglobin, packed cell volume, and hematocrit determinations are made.

Using 11 gm/100 ml hemoglobin (Hb) as the cutting point for diagnosis of anemia at this age, 37 percent of the infants were found to have anemia,[20] with 13.5 percent below 10 gm and 3.8 percent below 9 gm. While this is well below the rates of anemia in infants reported from other parts of Israel,[21] it does reflect that a mild degree of iron deficiency type anemia is common in this community, and more marked anemia is also found. There are differences by social class[22] and, as a result, between the three neighborhoods, the percentage of babies with anemia being 21, 38 and 52 in the middle-class, poor, and very poor neighborhoods, respectively. Sex was the other variable in which a highly significant association with hemoglobin was found, females having a higher mean hemoglobin.

As indicated above, the iron intake of these children as a whole is considerably below the United States RDA, and it is tempting to relate the anemia rate to a low iron intake. However, only a limited association between the total iron intake and anemia has been found in these babies. An interesting observation was an association between iron intake from heme sources and anemia, the higher the proportion of iron from heme sources as found at the 6 months dietary survey, the lower the prevalence of anemia at 9 months of age. This was in accord with the practice of earlier introduction of meat in infant feeding in the middle-class neighborhood than in the poorer localities. However, there was no association between iron intake from heme sources and social class, in children 30 to 48 months of age.

A second blood sample is taken at 24 months. The hemoglobin at this age is higher than that at 9 months, but differences in the anemia rate persist, 10 percent of middle-class children and 30 percent in the poorer neighborhoods.

In summary, the community diagnosis indicates an adequate, if not more than adequate, intake of nutrients, except for a possible deficiency in iron. The major inadequacy was that of breast feeding. Only 7 percent of the women interviewed were breast-feeding their babies at 6 months of age. There were differences between the mothers of different neighborhoods. A higher percentage of mothers living in the middle-class neighborhoods breast-fed their babies at birth, 1, 3, and 6 months than did those in the poor neighborhood, the respective figures being 82 : 69, 63 : 28, 17 : 7, and 8 : 3.

Differences in physical growth and in diet are not as marked as expected in babies of families with marked differences in social class and education. However, the higher percentage of low weight and short children in the poorer than in the middle-class neighborhoods suggests the need for action and continued monitoring. Similarly, the overweight children need attention.

The anemia rate in all groups, especially in the poorer neighborhoods, is in accord with expectations and led to a decision to intervene. The case for action is both an immediate one, focusing on a mild degree of malnutrition, and a more long-term need for surveillance, which will ensure early community diagnosis of a possible decline in health and growth in the light of the economic situation of the country. A rapid rise in the cost of foods as part of an inflationary spiral might adversely affect the poorer sections of the child population.

Psychomotor Development

One of the aims of community diagnosis of psychomotor development has been to determine the differential distribution of the Development Quotient (DQ) in various groups of the total infant population.[4,23] The

Brunet-Lezine test was used for assessing development, since it had previously been used in a study of Jerusalem children, and would thus allow for comparison.[24] The test is similar to the foundation of Gesell tests laid down many years ago, and consists of four component parts: language, postural-locomotor (gross motor), coordination-adaptation, and social-personal. The use of such a test for purposes of community diagnosis required standardization of methods in its application by primary care physicians and a psychologist, who were trained to carry it out. This standardization was done for the Brunet-Lezine tests at 9 and 24 months.

The community diagnosis focused on two major objectives of primary and secondary prevention:

1. To determine the frequency distribution of the DQ and its component parts, in the community of infants as a whole and in specially defined subgroups, according to ethnic origin, mother's educational standards, social class by father's occupational grade, and the baby's birth rank. In doing this, it was expected that we would be able to define subgroups of families in the population at risk for low DQ babies and thus in need of special attention.
2. To identify children having a low DQ score (below 80), or a low score in one of the component parts of the test. This screening procedure would lead to further investigation and, if necessary, referral to the child development center of Jerusalem.

The 9-month DQ test showed statistically significant differences in the total DQ score and in each subscore—social, language, postural, and coordination—by birth rank. Differences in the total DQ score were also found for birth weight, but not for mother's education and social class.

The test at 2 years of age also provided important information. Ethnic differences were marked. The children born to mothers from Europe or the Americas scored the highest mean DQ, and also the highest in language, posture, and coordination subscores. The lowest scores were attained by children whose mothers' origin was Africa or Asia, other than Israel. The Israeli group was a little behind those of Europe/America. However, these differences between ethnic groups were dependent on other factors.

Thus, the ethnic differences were not significant when analysis of variance was done, controlling for the age and education of the mother, social class, and birth order of the child. By contrast, when mother's education was similarly analyzed, controlling for the effects of the other four variables, significant differences were found in DQ as a whole, and especially in the language subscore. This finding is consistent with that of another investigation of Jerusalem children, in which parental education and the DQ of children aged 2 to 4 years were found to be associated.[24] The analysis also showed differences between children according to birth rank; the higher the rank, the lower the DQ and the language subscore. When controlling for the other four factors by analysis of variance, the difference remained statistically significant only for the language subscore.

This analysis has allowed for definition of the main family risk factors, namely, families with mothers of low educational standard (below 8 years) and large families with three or more children. As a result, the team decided to focus special attention on such families, with the objective of promoting higher than expected behavior development as measured by the DQ and its component parts.

INTERVENTION

Objectives of the intervention program are outlined in Figure 6–1, and include the promotion of physical growth, nutrition, behavioral and intellectual development, especially focused on infants of poor and uneducated families, by improving health, diet, social functioning, and protection against infection.

In considering the case for action, we need to relate the community diagnosis to what is already being done about the state of health and its determinants. When this program was initiated, we had evidence of marked differences in weight growth of infants and in the physique, especially height, of 3- and 4 year-olds between poorer and middle-class families. From the community diagnosis now emerging, this difference has been considerably reduced.

Among the factors responsible for this improvement is probably a decline in severer forms of gastroenteritis, and this may well be related to the widespread use of refrigerators, and hence more hygienic storage of milk, milk products, and other foods. Improving standards of education of mothers is probably a major factor for better nutrition, hygiene, and more effective response to the health education given by maternal and child health services. The dietary findings are indicative of the fact that the differences between children of different social classes are small. Similarly, protection against infection and secondary prevention of the ill effects of acute infectious illness are important existing assets. Thus, no statistically significant association has been found between anemia in infancy and the number of acute episodes of infectious illness for which medical

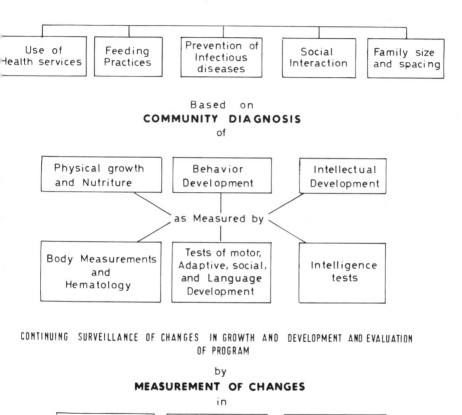

**PROMOTION OF
GROWTH AND DEVELOPMENT**

by

INVESTIGATION AND CHANGES OF BEHAVIOR WHERE NECESSARY IN

Use of Health services	Feeding Practices	Prevention of Infectious diseases	Social Interaction	Family size and spacing

Based on
COMMUNITY DIAGNOSIS
of

Physical growth and Nutriture	Behavior Development	Intellectual Development

as Measured by

Body Measurements and Hematology	Tests of motor, Adaptive, social, and Language Development	Intelligence tests

CONTINUING SURVEILLANCE OF CHANGES IN GROWTH AND DEVELOPMENT AND EVALUATION
OF PROGRAM

by
MEASUREMENT OF CHANGES
in

Growth	Behavior	Development

FIG. 6-1. Theoretic model of program for promotion of growth and development (PROD).

care was sought.[25] Perhaps this is evidence of a moderately good nutritional status associated with resistance to infection, as well as effective treatment of infectious illness. Surveillance of infectious illness has recently been included in the PROD program; a record is made of illness occurrence at 3-month intervals through infancy.

What then remains to be done? When we started this program the case for action was clear, but the differences in physical growth in various social groups that was apparent in the 1960s has narrowed considerably. There is no case at this time for a major community program directed to change in growth by diet and nutrition. Ways of encouraging breast-feeding need further serious consideration. At present, the main focus is on a program concerned with treatment of anemia, and another on promoting behavioral development through increased social interaction, including verbal stimulation and play.

The Control of Anemia in Infancy

The main somatic defect requiring further attention is that of anemia in infancy, and for this a program is now being carried out as an integral part of the maternal and child health services of the health center. The examination procedure and the findings have been previously outlined.

For purposes of this program, any infant with a hemoglobin level below 11 gm/100 ml is regarded as a case of anemia in need of treatment. This follows the recommendation of a technical committee of the World Health Organization on nutritional anemia.[20] Following a diagnosis of anemia at 9 months of age, the treatment consists of 4 percent ferrous sulphate syrup, three times daily, for a daily total of between 5 and 7.5 cc. The treatment continues for at least 2 months, when a further blood specimen is examined. Associated with this secondary prevention objective is a reinforcement of the health education program on infant feeding, with special attention to breast-feeding and the desirability of foods containing iron from heme sources, such as liver and other meats. Iron supplementation is given to all LBW (2500 gm and below) babies through the first year of life.

Early results of this treatment were encouraging[21] in that the response rate was in accord with the degree of anemia. The blood tests were repeated on the treated children between 12 and 15 months. Seventy babies with an initial hemoglobin level of 10 to 10.9 had an average increase of 1.4 gm/100 ml, whereas the average increase in 25 babies with level 9 to 9.9 was 2.5, and the seven cases below this figure responded with an average increase of more than 4 gm/100 ml. The net effect at the end of treatment was to equalize the hemoglobin levels of the previously anemic babies in the middle-class, poor, and very poor areas, namely, 12.1, 12.0, and 12.0 gm/100 ml.

The Promotion of Behavior Development

The program introduced at the health center is based on an approach developed by Ortar.[26] Following observations of various groups of mothers talking with their children, she established a program to teach mothers to speak to their children in ways that would promote verbal development. Relative backwardness in verbal development of children has been linked with lack of verbal interaction between mothers and their babies. Thus, in a study of a particular culture group in Israel, it was found that young children were not often spoken to except on basic matters and they were not stimulated to develop their vocabulary or to ask questions.[27]

We felt that programs of the kind developed in the United States[28-31] and in Israel, adapted to the primary care situation in which mother and nurse are discussing the baby's progress, would be feasible in our practice. Ortar was invited to demonstrate her method to the health center staff. The nurses were guided to incorporate into their routine work ways of teaching mothers how to speak to their babies in order to promote enriching speech.

In the same way as the mother-child record includes guides to feeding at different ages, weight and height standards, and developmental records, a special form has been included in the file, listing items that the nurse advises the mother to do. These activities, verbal and toy playing, are arranged according to the age at which the child should be exposed to them. In the first 2 months, these activities include such items as having the child listen to songs, talking to the baby while doing daily activities, calling the child by name, talking to him or her from a distance, and playing with or looking at mobiles and room decorations. By the age of 1 year, the step-by-step program guide includes imitation of words and word combinations, telling the child short stories, encouraging communication between baby and other people, playing hide-and-seek, providing pulling toys, and building towers of blocks. Until recently, this has been done through the first year of the child's life, but has since been extended with the use of an additional guide prepared for the ages 1 through 3 years.

The introduction of such a program into the routine work of a nurse in a mother and child care clinic may present problems. It is so unlike the usual activities of nurses, even those involved with preventive work, that resistance may be expected from a number of them. With patient, persistent in-service training, this has been changed. This is a first level of evaluation of a program, namely, are we ourselves doing what we set out to do?

Can similar programs be introduced into the routines of nonteaching maternal and child health centers? The answer is yes. They are extending to other centers in the country. By arrangement with the City Health department of Jerusalem, the PROD team has introduced a modified program into a maternal and child health center of an adjacent area of Kiryat Yovel. Measurements of physical growth and DQ are conducted. The program for the control of anemia, and that of verbal stimulation and play activity, have been successfully incorporated.

Other activities by the PROD team have included group sessions with mothers at their homes, focusing on verbal stimulation and play. The knowledge of mothers in these groups was significantly improved when compared with a control group.[32] Another program is that of a community center, which is adjacent to our departmental health center. An intensive play-care program for selected 2- to 4-year-olds has been in progress since 1976. Evaluation of this program is being conducted by the director of the PROD program, who reports encouraging trends.

Evaluation of effectiveness of the overall program is being carried out, using the DQ test findings at 24 months, and will also be made by using measurements of intelligence at 3 and 5 years. The latter is being done on children as they enter the compulsory nursery school year, before attending regular first grade. The children included in this PROD program are now reaching this age. Some of the problems of such evaluation are discussed further.

EVALUATION OF THE PROD PROGRAM: SOME PROBLEMS

The maternal and child health service of the health center now includes a well-established community program focused on growth and development, nutrition and dietary practices, immunization, family planning, and promotion of development by verbal stimulation and play. At the same time as these developments are taking place in expanding the practice of health care, other social and demographic changes are occurring, which make it difficult to evaluate the effect of the health program itself. Among the more important of these in Kiryat Yovel have been movement of the population, improvement in the standard of living, and decrease in the size of the family.

Geographic mobility has been of two kinds. There has been considerable mobility of young adults in Kiryat Yovel. Thus, there is a continuing inward movement of young couples, especially university students, who on completion of their studies leave the area for other parts of Jerusalem or elsewhere in the country. Migration data for the various census tracts included in Kiryat Yovel show that slightly over half of all movement in and out of the area occurred in the age group 15 to 29. Between 25 and 30 percent of this age group migrate each year, with approximately equal numbers moving in and out of the area. The influence of this on continuity of care of infants and young children wil be readily appreciated. Thus, of 110 children in one birth cohort who were examined at 18 months, there were only 75 available for examination at 4 years, the remainder having moved away.[16] Nevertheless, it is important to note that 68 percent of the children were still living in the neighborhood.

Another movement of population has affected one whole neighborhood of Kiryat Yovel. During the years since this program was initiated, a poor neighborhood consisting of temporary huts has steadily been demolished, and the families have been transferred to better housing in other parts of the city. There are now very few families with infants and young children in this area, a neighborhood that housed more than 2000 people including a number of children who were in the main target group of PROD. The decline of this population has removed a number of children from the program.

The high rate of mobility of young families, coupled with the rehousing program, cause considerable problems for the continuity of care required by this kind of long-term, community-oriented, health program. However, despite these difficulties, there is a substantial core of families who remain in the area, often in the same homes, and they do have the opportunity for continuity in their participation in the program.

In addition to geographic mobility, there are other problems in attempting evaluation of a program such as PROD. These include an improved standard of living, upward social mobility, and reduction in family size. Along with the rest of the country, there has been social, economic, and educational advance in Kiryat Yovel. This is especially noticeable in the decline of the proportion of the population in the lower socioeconomic classes and those with a very low standard of education. The mothers of today's children are better educated than those of the last generation, which is perhaps the most striking feature in the upward social mobility of the people in this area. Associated with this has been a decline in the birth rate and size of family, with a consequent lower proportion of high birth rank children, a particularly susceptible group at risk for developmental retardation. The combined influence of these social changes would lead us to expect a lessening of differences in growth and development of infants and young children in the families of different social and economic status in this community.

Originally it had been planned to include several control communities, in which general medical care and well-child health services were readily available. A number of centers were selected in consultation with those responsible for the local services. However, although the services were accessible, they were insufficiently utilized to be useful as control populations. It would have demanded intensive additional activity, including home visits, to raise the level of attendance needed. This itself would have a nonmeasurable effect on this population, thereby vitiating its value as a control group in an evaluation study.

CONCLUSION

In most countries that have a well-developed maternal and child health service, child health care as distinct from medical care of sick children is not an integral part of the functions of primary care physicians, more especially the general practitioner/family physician or pediatrician. This is also true in Israel, where the network of maternal and child health centers of the country are, in the main, separate from the medical insurance clinics of Kupat Holim. These latter are usually curative clinics. This means that medical insurance, which provides ready access to medical care of sick children, does not, in itself, ensure the basic elements of promotive and preventive child health care. As we have seen, special provision has been made for this. The Kupat Holim, which has the responsibility for conducting a number of maternal and child health centers, is moving toward an integration of these services into a number of their clinics. They are using different methods. One of the major problems in such integration is the priority often given to the needs of the sick at the expense of promotive and preventive care.

In reviewing differences in child health and social programs in the United States and six European countries, Silver[33] reaches certain conclusions that are not only relevant to our present discussion, but demand the attention of all who are concerned with child health and welfare. He finds that eligibility for medical care, per se, does not guarantee preventive services for children and that preventive services are not only desirable, but necessary. He regards specially trained child health nurses as a key factor for high quality of such services.

While we agree that special provision needs to be made to ensure delivery of preventive services, no case is made for continuing with the separation of the various primary care services. There are, in fact, a number of voices in favor of some such addition to the functions of primary medical care carried out by physicians. Thus in the United Kingdom, the Court Report on Child Health Services recommends that child health care, including the surveillance of health and development, should be carried out within the framework of general practice.[34] It recognizes that this would require special training of large numbers of general practitioners in that country and recommends that this be done. While there has been some resistance to the proposals on the part of many general practitioners, there are positive responses. Surveillance and screening of child development by general practitioners has been reported.[35] This may be a beginning of the integration of preventive functions into the practice of primary care physicians.

Much attention continues to be focused on child health, and the need for widening the perspective in which child health care should be considered. And rightly so, since at the same time technology and its use in hospitals continues to use the main financial and manpower resources available. The assumptions behind this need to be challenged and have been by many outstanding workers. In a comprehensive review of child health in America,[36] Newberger, Newberger, and Richmond question premises such as the belief that advances in technical methods ensure the control of illness, that health care for children consists of immunizations and intervention in acute illness, that the provision of services ensures their equitable use, and that the best health service is that provided by physicians. In a carefully annotated review, they discredit these beliefs and provide a detailed outline of proposals that emphasize promotive and preventive aspects and the need for planning of child health care along with other child care services.

One of the interesting features of child health care is the difference in its organization in various countries. The reasons may be historical-social, or they may be a reflection of different objectives and orientations. Although the differences may be suited to the various settings, it is perhaps useful and expedient to consider further the objectives and orientation of society's provisions for health and well-being of children.

Objectives.   The objectives of child health care may be considered comprehensively as consisting of the following elements:

Promotion of Health and Well-Being.   An example is a program for the promotion of child growth and development, such as that outlined in the review of PROD. Similar promotive programs might be centered on health education for the improvement of nutritional status or emotional health of children, or on social action other than health services, such as the latent health functions of schools and sporting activities.

Prevention and Protection from Disease and Injury.   This includes well-established procedures of immunization against infectious disease, protection from infection by food, environmental sanitation, and the inculcation of hygienic personal habits. It also includes protection against child abuse and other social pathologies.

Treatment and Alleviation of Illness and Disability.   The aspect with which we are mainly concerned here is the curative practice of primary health care, which should be coordinated with that of hospitals and other secondary and tertiary care institutions.

Rehabilitation.   This involves the special measures, educational, social, psychologic, and physical, which are needed to help develop the abilities of handicapped children. It has application to mental or physical causes of disability, whether congenital or acquired.

Orientation.   The orientation of different elements of the health system may be toward the individual patient only, to the individual and family, or to the community as a whole and its subgroups. Much primary health care is centered on individual children, the medical care of sick children being an obvious example. Even preventive services for children are often focused on the individual child in the family, with the public health nurse concerned with family and home as they affect the child. The question raised in this chapter on a community program for the promotion of growth and development (PROD) is whether the focus on the individual child in the family would be improved by an orientation extending to the community as a whole. Acceptance of responsibility for the well-being of the child population in a community goes beyond the care of children who turn to a health facility for advice and care. It extends to those for whom mothers do not seek care, recognizing, as did the pioneers of the child health movement in Europe and the United States, that such children may be most in need of society's interest and concern.

Hospital medicine has led to almost complete orientation to the individual patient, and the teaching hospital as part of medical schools has intensified this to exclusive concern with the clinical-pathologic aspects of care. This process of professional socialization has, at the same time, directed the interest and skills of the dominant health profession, medicine, away from the social aspects of child health, more especially family- and community-oriented health care.

Organization. The organization of child health care may only partly reflect the objectives and orientation of such care. The common separation of curative, preventive, and welfare services should not in itself preclude a community orientation. The three primary services may be integrated into the functions of a single health team, or they may continue as separate primary care services, providing they have adequate links with one another and coordinate their activities in respect of individuals, families, and the child community as a whole. If their functions are brought together by a single health team, it is important to specify the promotive, preventive, and welfare objectives, in addition to the curative, and to train members of the health team to fulfill the functions required to attain these objectives.

The case, illustrated here by PROD, is that community-oriented primary health care has universal application as a model for primary care. It is feasible to develop it in the framework of integrated services or in separately provided services. The focus might be on different priorities. Thus, in an area with high mortality rates or special morbidity problems, such as hookworm infestation, protein-calorie malnutrition, or lead poisoning, the community program would include focus on one of these. It is to the use of primary health care as a vehicle of public health that this chapter on community-oriented primary health care of children is addressed.

REFERENCES

1. Statistical Abstract of Israel. Jerusalem, Central Bureau of Statistics, 1979
2. Epstein LM: Growth in weight of infants in the western region of Jerusalem, Israel. J Trop Pediatr 14:139, 1968
3. Flug D: Height and weight growth of children in two different neighborhoods. Cited in Kark SL: Epidemiology and Community Medicine. New York, Appleton, 1974, p 416
4. Kark SL: A community program for promotion of growth and development. In Kark SL: Epidemiology and Community Medicine. New York, Appleton, 1974, p 415
5. Lieblich A, Ninio A, Kugelmass S: Effects of ethnic origin and parental SES on WPPSI performance of pre-schoolchildren in Israel. J Cross-Cultural Psychol 3:159, 1972
6. Ortar G: A comparative analysis of the structure of intelligence in various ethnic groups. In Frankenstein C (ed): Between Past and Future—Essays and Studies on Aspects of Immigrant Absorption in Israel. Jerusalem, Henrietta Szold Foundation for Child and Youth Welfare, 1953, p 267

7. ———: Educational achievements of primary school graduates in Israel as related to their socioeconomic background. Comp Educ 4:23, 1967

8. Clarke AM, Clarke ADB (eds): Mental Deficiency: The Changing Outlook. London, Methuen, 1958

9. Stein Z, Susser MW: The social distribution of mental retardation. Am J Ment Defic 67:811, 1963

10. Susser MW: Community Psychiatry. New York, Random House, 1968

11. Richardson SA: The influence of socioenvironmental and nutritional factors on mental ability. In Scrimshaw NS, Gordon JE (eds): Malnutrition, Learning and Behavior. Cambridge, MIT Press, 1968

12. National Center for Health Statistics: Intellectual Development and School Achievement of Youths 12–17 years: Demographic and Socioeconomic Factors. United States. Vital and Health Statistics Series 11 No. 158. DHEW Publication No. (HRA) 77.1640, 1976

13. Brunet O, Lezine I: Le Développement Psychologique de l'Enfant. Paris, Presses Universitaires de France, 1951

14. Ortar G, Hagari A, Kartony-Makov H: "M.I.L.I." Intelligence Scale for Preschool Children, Age 3–6 years. Jerusalem, School of Education, Hebrew University and Ministry of Education and Culture, 1966

15. Palti H, Adler B, Reshef A: A semilongitudinal study of food intake, anemia rate, and body measurements of 6- to 24-month-old children in a Jerusalem community. Am J Clin Nutr 30:268, 1977

16. Palti H, Reshef A, Adler B: Food intake and growth of children between 30 and 48 months of age in Jerusalem. Pediatrics 63:713, 1979

17. National Center for Health Statistics: Growth Curves for Children Birth–18 Years. United States. Vital and Health Statistics. Series 11 No. 165. DHEW Publication No. (PHS) 78–1650, 1977

18. National Research Council: Recommended Dietary Allowances. Washington, D.C., National Academy of Sciences, 8th rev. ed., 1974

19. Passmore R, Nicol BM, Rao MN: Handbook on Human Nutritional Requirements. Geneva, WHO, 1974

20. World Health Organization: Nutritional Anemias. Technical Report Series No. 503, Geneva, WHO, 1972

21. Palti H, Gitlin M, Shamir Z: Anemia in infancy. A community program of surveillance and evaluation of treatment (in Hebrew with English summary). Harefuah 92:69, 1976

22. Palti H, Adler B, Wolf N: An epidemiological study of hemoglobin levels in infancy in Jerusalem. Acta Paediatr Scand 66:513, 1977

23. ———, Adler B, Flug D, et al.: Community diagnosis of psychomotor development in infancy. Isr Ann Psychiatry 15:223, 1977

24. Smilansky S, Shephatia L, Frenkel E: Mental Development of Infants from Two Ethnic Groups. Research Report No. 195. Jerusalem, Henrietta Szold Institute. The National Institute for Research in the Behavioral Sciences, 1976

25. Palti H, Zloto R, Gampel B: Infection rate and anemia in infancy in a Jerusalem community. Isr J Med Sci 15:165, 1979

26. Ortar G, Carmon H: An Analysis of Mother's Speech as a Factor in the Development of Children's Intelligence. (Mimeograph Report) Jerusalem, Hebrew Univ. School of Education, 1969

27. Weintraub D, Shapiro M: The family in process of change. In Weintraub D (ed): Immigration and Social Change. Jerusalem, Israel Univ. Press, and Manchester, Manchester Univ. Press, 1971, p 166

28. Gordon J, Guinagh B, Jester RE: Child Learning Through Child Play. New York, St Martin's, 1972
29. Gordon J: Baby Learning Through Baby Play. New York, St Martin's, 1970
30. Levenstein P: Verbal Interaction Project. Freeport, N.Y., Mother-Child Home Program, mimeograph material, 1977
31. Levenstein P: Model Programs. Compensatory Education. Washington, D.C., DHEW Publication No. (OE) 72–84, 1972
32. Feigenbaum J: Knowledge and Attitudes of Mothers in Western Jerusalem Towards Infant Verbal and Play Development. Jerusalem, Master of Public Health Dissertation. Department of Social Medicine, Hebrew University-Hadassah Medical School, 1978
33. Silver GA: Some observations on preventive health services for children. European and American policies and programs. Courrier 28: 233, 1978
34. Committee on Child Health Services: Fit for the Future. Court Report. London, HMSO, 1976
35. Jenkins GHC, Collins C, Andrew S: Developmental surveillance in general practice. Br Med J I:1537, 1978
36. Newberger EH, Newberger CM, Richmond JB: Child Health in America: toward a rational public policy. Health and Society. Milbank Mem Fund Q 54:249, 1976

CHAPTER 7

COMMUNITY MEDICINE IN THE PRIMARY HEALTH CARE OF URBAN ADULTS

THE CONTROL OF A COMMUNITY SYNDROME OF HYPERTENSION, ATHEROSCLEROTIC DISEASES, AND DIABETES (CHAD)

A major public health problem in many countries is presented by the concurrent prevalence of a group of circulatory and metabolic disorders. These include ischemic heart disease, hypertensive heart disease and renal disease, cerebrovascular disease, peripheral vascular disease, hypertension, diabetes mellitus and hyperglycemia, and hyperlipidemia. It is the co-prevalence of these conditions that is of special interest in the present context, and we refer to it as CHAD, a community syndrome of hypertension, atherosclerotic diseases, and diabetes mellitus.[1] Their interaction with one another has been the subject of many studies and has established some of the factors as being risk factors for others. Thus, high blood pressure and hypercholesterolemia occurring together are risk factors for ischemic heart disease, and in this context, persons with diabetes mellitus are at considerably greater risk for ischemic heart disease.[2-6] There has been a steady increase in understanding some of the determinants, such as genetic and life experience, especially diet and nutrition, cigarette smoking, personality, and precipitating factors such as life crises.

In 1970, when we planned to initiate a program for the control and prevention of the CHAD conditions, the case for action was clear. Over the previous 20 years, there had been a rise in the death rate from ischemic heart disease in Israel, especially in several of the immigrant communities, whose life style had changed considerably after their arrival in the country during this period. In the late 1960s, of all deaths in men and women 25 years and over in Israel, 59 percent were listed as due to cardiovascular diseases. Ischemic heart disease alone accounted for 34 percent of the male deaths and 28 percent of the female deaths; the corresponding proportions of adult deaths due to cerebrovascular disease were 15 and 14 percent.[7] Thus, Israel was increasingly coming to resemble a number of the more developed countries, with a high death rate from ischemic heart disease and cerebrovascular disease. There was also a high rate of several of the risk factors known to be associated with these fatal diseases, such as hypertension, hypercholesterolemia, hyperglycemia, and diabetes mellitus.

The annual food balance sheet published by the Central Bureau of Statistics of Israel reflects the probable changes in diet in the country over the past 30 years.[8] There has been an increase in several items that are of interest in the present context. From the year 1949–1950 to that of 1976–1977, the availability of calories, protein, and fat to the consumer has increased as follows:

Calories by more than 300 per capita per day, from 2610 to 3043.

Protein by more than 13 gm per capita per day, from 83.9 to 97.4.

Fat by more than 36 gm per capita per day, from 73.9 to 112.5.

The major feature of these changes has been the increase in the amount of meat, including poultry, accompanied by consistently high amounts of milk, milk products, and eggs. Sugar consumption increased in the first decade or more following the establishment of the state, and has since declined slightly from its peak.

With the increase in animal foods and sugar until 15 to 20 years ago, there has been a decline in the contribution of cereals and cereal products to the food balance sheet.

These factors and supporting data have been previously reported in considering the case for action of the CHAD program.[1]

We wished to test the feasibility and effectiveness of carrying out a program directed toward control of this community syndrome by a multifactorial approach within a primary care practice.

AIMS OF THE PROGRAM

The program was initiated in 1971 with the general aim of reducing the risk factors for hypertension and ischemic heart disease, cerebrovascular disease, and peripheral vascular disease within the framework of a general family practice by implementing the following:

1. The establishment of a health team, consisting of members of the department of social medicine and the health center, which would develop a program in the framework of the family practice of the departmental health center in Kiryat Yovel.
2. A trial of feasibility in the use of primary health care as an important vehicle in meeting a major public health problem.
3. Setting up methods for community diagnosis and ongoing surveillance of the relevant health conditions and their determinants.
4. Where necessary and possible, development of intervention programs, in order to achieve the following:
   a. Change in the community distribution of blood pressure levels, serum cholesterol, serum glucose, and relative weight.
   b. Screening of cases with hypertension, hypercholesterolemia, obesity, and cigarette smoking, with the objectives of treating and counseling affected individuals and thereby reducing the prevalence of these risk factors.
   c. Similarly, identification and treatment of cases with the circulatory diseases listed above, and diabetes mellitus.
   d. Encouragement of community response to use of the health services, and if necessary, carrying out of medicinal treatment advised or modification of diet, exercise, and smoking habits.
5. Evaluation of the program, including each of its various components.

A summary of the elements of the CHAD program is shown in Figure 7-1.

THE HEALTH TEAM

The early development of the CHAD program was the responsibility of a special team, composed of epidemiologists, family physicians, a specialist physician in nutrition, community health nurses, community health workers, a statistician-health recorder, and a social psychiatrist. The members of this team met frequently and were responsible for detailed planning, work assignments, and the direction of the program. Progress in planning and action was reported to the

CASE FINDING AND TREATMENT
of

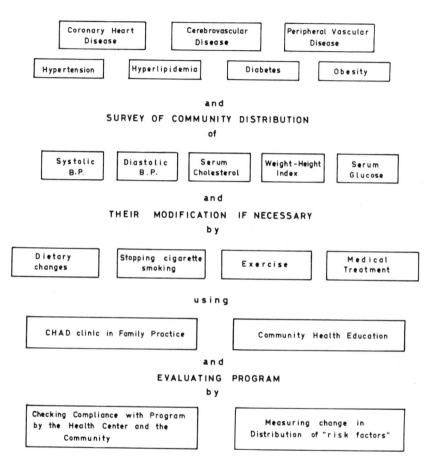

| Coronary Heart Disease | Cerebrovascular Disease | Peripheral Vascular Disease |

| Hypertension | Hyperlipidemia | Diabetes | Obesity |

and
SURVEY OF COMMUNITY DISTRIBUTION
of

| Systolic B.P. | Diastolic B.P. | Serum Cholesterol | Weight-Height Index | Serum Glucose |

and
THEIR   MODIFICATION   IF NECESSARY
by

| Dietary changes | Stopping cigarette smoking | Exercise | Medical Treatment |

using

| CHAD clinic in Family Practice | Community Health Education |

and
EVALUATING   PROGRAM
by

| Checking Compliance with Program by the Health Center and the Community | Measuring change in Distribution of "risk factors" |

FIG. 7-1. Summary of the elements of the CHAD program. [From Kark, 1974 (see Ref. 1).]

group conference of staff members of the department of social medicine and the health center at the weekly community medicine round (CMR).

The functions of the different members of the CHAD team are described here in relation to the three constituent elements of the health team outlined in Chapter 3: the family practice team members, the team members with special skills for community medicine programs, and consultants for special aspects of the CHAD program.

Family Practice Team Members

The feasibility of integrating a community medicine program, such as CHAD, within the framework of primary health care is a major objective of the project. High priority has been given to defining and developing the roles of different members of the family practice team in carrying out the program, especially the family physicians and nurses. From the outset, the family physicians were involved in decision making about the general and detailed objectives, the methods to be used, and the division of functions of different members. In addition, they had direct responsibility in carrying out the program. Each person's record was reviewed by the team, a proposed program was agreed upon, and special appointments were made for the individuals or family members concerned, for discussion of the findings and suggested action.

The introduction of the CHAD program to the family nurses was different from that of the family physicians. The chief nurse of the family practice team was an early member of the team involved at all levels of decision making about the program. She felt that for the proper integration of such a community medicine program into the family practice, each family nurse would need to have responsibility for the individuals and families in the geographic area for which she was responsible. Following special training of the family nurses for their role in CHAD, they now share in the responsibility for carrying out the program.

Members with Special Skills
in Community Medicine

Epidemiology and Biostatistics. Ensuring that the program is based on sound epidemiologic methods is the function of epidemiologists and statisticians of the department of social medicine. They have been involved in planning of the program and its execution, which includes community diagnosis, ongoing surveillance of health, the intervention program, and evaluation of the program.

Initially, the program was directed by an epidemiologist. This is now the responsibility of one of the senior family physicians.

Special Community Nurse. In addition to the chief nurse of the family practice, another family and community nurse was a foundation member of the CHAD team. She had considerable experience in health surveys, especially as the nurse organizer of a community health survey, and contributed much to the planning and decision making of the team.

The special community nurse continues to function as a coordinator, ensuring that the total program is being carried out by various members of the team.

Community Organization and Health Education. An important member of the health center team is a community organizer/health educator, who has had graduate training in both community organization and public health. His specific role in this program was as one of the team members introducing the community to the program. He met with various groups within the community, religious, ethnic, political, and informal leaders, all of whom responded very positively to involvement in such a community project.

Consultants

Consultative functions are both clinical and community oriented. The ways in which clinical consultations are carried out vary from referral of a patient in this practice to a hospital or another service, clinical consultations at the health center itself or at the home of a housebound patient, for example by a physiotherapist or occupational therapist.

The various units of the department of social medicine act as consultants to the overall program. The roles such consultants have played in the CHAD program have included the active participation by a physician specialist in public health nutrition and discussions of different elements of the program with internists and others about the management of such conditions as diabetes mellitus and essential hypertension.

Supportive Members of the Team

Supportive members of the team are those whose functions flow from the needs of the community-oriented primary care team. For example, the recording system of the practice is an essential supportive service which, with the introduction of community medicine within the primary care practice, needed modification to meet the requirements of individual and family records, and community diagnosis, surveillance, and evaluation. In fact, the chief of the health records section in the health center is a key member of the CHAD team, both in her role as director of the health records and as a biostatistician, having special skills in the use of statistics in community medicine programs such as CHAD.

COMMUNITY DIAGNOSIS
AND HEALTH SURVEILLANCE

The initial community diagnosis was based on data from two main sources. When we started the CHAD program, we had almost completed a community health survey (1969–1971) of all the adults, and 50 percent of the children, living in a defined geographic area of Kiryat Yovel, with an estimated total population of 10,000, of whom some 3000 lived in the defined area of our family practice.[9] The findings of this community health survey, together with data extracted from each individual's clinical records at the health center, served as the baseline information for the initial community diagnosis. The data required for this community diagnosis, and subsequent surveillance, were related to:

Diagnoses of ischemic heart disease, cerebrovascular disease, and peripheral vascular disease, as well as other diseases.
Blood pressure and hypertension.
Cholesterol levels and hyperlipidemia.
Uric acid levels, hyperuricemia, and gout.
Blood sugar levels, hyperglycemia, and diabetes mellitus.
Weight, height, and obesity.
Diet, cigarette smoking, physical exercise, and medications being taken.

Special records were designed for the extraction of data from the community health survey and the clinical records of the family practice. Data on each person examined during the community health survey were abstracted onto a special CHAD record form, and the relevant findings from the records of the family practice were then summarized on this special form. This provided data needed for preliminary epidemiologic analysis of the distribution by age and sex of various diseases and risk factors. By studying these two sets of findings together, we were able to classify each individual according to the highest risk reading ever recorded. We realized that this would result in the inclusion of a number of false positives, but felt this to be desirable for our initial scoring of those considered to be in need of further investigation.

There were 956 people aged 25 years and over in the family practice, who were examined in the community health survey. The combined findings of the clinical records and community health survey in respect of blood pressure, serum cholesterol, serum glucose, and relative weight were among the initial data examined (Table 7–1).

TABLE 7-1

**The Percentage Distribution of Various Risk Factors in 956 Men and Women
According to Age, in the Family Practice of the
Kiryat Yovel Health Center 1969-1971***

	25-44 YEARS		45-64 YEARS		65 YEARS +	
	Men	Women	Men	Women	Men	Women
mber in group	187	238	152	195	85	99
k Factor Level						
stolic BP (mm/Hg)						
3orderline 140-159	18.2	15.5	28.3	30.8	24.7	15.2
ligh 160+	4.3	7.2	36.8	50.8	65.9	78.8
astolic BP (mm/Hg)						
3orderline 90-94	18.2	13.4	15.8	21.0	25.9	10.1
ligh 95+	11.2	11.8	46.7	50.3	47.1	70.7
rum cholesterol (mg/100ml)						
3orderline 200-239	27.8	31.5	30.9	27.7	37.6	26.3
ligh 240+	11.2	14.7	45.4	55.4	38.8	65.7
um glucose (mg/100ml)						
3orderline 180 or						
ossible diabetes						
mellitus	5.3	3.8	9.9	11.3	9.4	13.1
ligh: Diagnosis of dia-						
etes mellitus	1.1	2.5	17.1	11.8	23.5	25.3
ative weight						
3orderline: 10-19 per-						
ent above standard						
veight	19.3	21.4	23.0	20.5	22.4	13.1
ligh: 20+ percent						
bove standard weight	12.8	29.0	28.9	52.8	16.5	50.5

or criteria and explanatory notes see text and Reference 10.

These risk factors commonly occur together in this community, especially in the middle-aged and older people.

Blood Pressure and Hypertension

Defining the Risk Status of Individuals.   The first screening of hypertension cases was based on the findings of the community health survey and the clinical records of the individuals at the health center (Fig. 7-1). All persons with a highest ever recorded blood pressure level of 140 mm Hg or over systolic, and/or 90 mm Hg or over diastolic, were invited for furthor oxaminatious in order to assess their blood pressure status and commence treatment or surveillance, depending on the assessment. Of the total 956 adults in the family practice, aged 25 years and over who were examined in the community health study, 345 individuals (31 percent) were thus assessed. In doubtful cases, ten successive readings within 1 month were initially required. This has since been reduced to three successive readings, which were found to yield the same results.

Within approximately a year of the initiation of the program, 73 percent (253) of those initially screened were examined, with the following results:

	Number	Percent
Normal blood pressure (systolic below 140 and diastolic below 90)	65	25.7
Borderline blood pressure (systolic 140–159 and/or diastolic 90–94)	83	32.8
High blood pressure (systolic 160 or over and/ or diastolic 95 or over)	105	41.5

The false-positive rate in these 253 cases was thus 25.7 percent, and 41.5 percent needed treatment. Hypertension was common in both men and women.

Blood Pressure by Age and Sex.   In order to have a wider perspective in making our community diagnosis, the blood pressure data of the total population examined in the community health survey are presented. This population, composed of some 5000 men and women, included the 956 in the family practice. The means and standard deviations have been analyzed by 10-year age groups for each sex (Table 7-2). As in the majority of world communities, this is one in which there is a rise in blood pressure with age in both sexes. The rise is noted in both men and women, being especially marked in respect of systolic blood pressure from the age of 45 years onward. The men have higher mean systolic blood pressure than the women in the younger age groups; the two groups are similar in the age groups 35 to 54; and in the older ages (55 and over), women are higher than the men. The sex differences in diastolic blood pressure are less marked, men being somewhat higher from 25 through to 54, after which there is little or no difference.

TABLE 7-2

The Mean Blood Pressure* in Men and Women, by Age Group

	AGE						
	15-24	25-34	35-44	45-54	55-64	65-74	75+
Number of Males	357	623	442	303	324	158	47
Systolic BP							
Mean	125.6	123.1	125.4	130.9	140.7	147.1	160.6
S.D.	14.9	14.2	16.4	20.3	25.2	24.4	29.2
Diastolic BP							
Mean	69.5	74.5	80.1	83.7	85.6	83.2	81.3
S.D.	12.3	11.4	12.2	12.9	14.5	13.5	17.8
Number of Females	541	724	477	390	311	160	66
Systolic BP							
Mean	116.3	114.3	122.0	132.5	147.8	155.4	168.0
S.D.	12.3	13.3	18.4	23.9	25.6	27.0	31.5
Diastolic BP							
Mean	70.4	70.4	76.9	81.0	85.9	84.6	87.0
S.D.	11.1	11.0	12.7	14.0	13.8	14.2	17.4

*Given in mm Hg.

Serum Cholesterol

Defining the Risk Status of Individuals.   All individuals in the family practice population with casual serum cholesterol levels of 240 mg/100 ml and over were classified as high-risk cases, and those with levels 200 to 239 as borderline risk (Table 7-1). The percentages of younger men and women, 25 to 44 years, who had a serum cholesterol level of 240 and over were 11 and 15, respectively. There was a sharp increase in the middle-aged men and women, 45 and 55 percent, respectively. In older women, 65 years and over, there is an even higher proportion above this level, 66 percent, but in men there is a decline to 39 percent.

Mean Serum Cholesterol by Age and Sex.   In the same way as was done for blood pressure, the mean serum cholesterol levels at different ages for the total population of 5000 men and women in the community health survey is presented in Table 7-3. The mean serum cholesterol level increases with each decade of age from 15 to 24 through to 74 in the men and 64 in the women, after which there is a slight decline. The steady rise with age and the actual high level at all ages are indicative of a need for intervention.

TABLE 7-3

The Mean Serum Cholesterol* In Mon and Women by Age Group

	AGE						
	15–24	25–34	35–44	45–54	55–64	65–74	75 +
Male							
Mean	165.8	191.9	211.6	215.7	220.3	223.4	213.5
S.D.	28.2	56.2	53.6	42.1	45.4	47.0	44.0
Female							
Mean	176.4	193.1	206.3	227.0	237.6	234.2	232.8
S.D.	34.3	39.3	35.8	47.2	46.0	40.7	48.7

*Given in mg/100 ml.

Diabetes Mellitus

All known diabetic cases were included in the initial list of those at risk. In addition, all others were given a screening test, 75-gm glucose drink under nonfasting conditions; a serum glucose level of 180 mg/100 ml or more, 1 hour later, was regarded as a positive indication for a subsequent glucose tolerance test (GTT). Following the GTT, the population was classified as normal, possible, probable, or definite.[1] The probable and definite cases, taken together with those already known to the family practice, were classified as diabetes mellitus.

In the family practice population, a marked rise in the proportion of persons diagnosed to have diabetes mellitus occurs in the middle age group, 45 to 64, from 1 to 17 percent in men and 3 to 12 percent in women. The rise continues, and in those over 65 years of age one in four men and women were diagnosed as diabetic (Table 7-1). The very high risk that diabetics have for cardiovascular disease is well known and is illustrated in the association of diabetes with hypertension, obesity, and cardiovascular diseases in the family practice population.[1]

Overweight

We classified the men and women in the family practice population according to the standard weight for height and sex, at age 25, as published by the U.S. Society of Actuaries.[11] Those found to be 20 percent above the standard weight for height were classified as overweight, those 10 to 19 percent above as borderline overweight, and those less than 10 percent above as normal. The three main age groups in the family practice population had a high proportion of overweight persons, among the men the 25 to 44, 45 to 64, and 65 and over age groups had 13, 29, and 16 percent who were 20 percent or more above the standard weight; a greater proportion of the women, 29, 53, and 50 percent in these age groups were in the overweight category.

Cigarette Smoking

The extent of cigarette smoking was determined in the community health survey. The heaviest smokers in the family practice population were the men aged 25 to 44 years, 57 percent being smokers, with 30 percent heavy smokers, that is, 20 cigarettes or more daily. Smoking by women of the same age group was also common, the corresponding figures being 34 and 10 percent. With increase in age, the prevalence of cigarette smoking declined in both sexes, but in the middle age group of 45 to 64 years, 46 percent of men and 22 percent of women smoked, with 16 and 6 percent, respectively, being classified as heavy smokers. Thus, the task ahead of the CHAD program was, and still is, considerable.

The Prevalence of Ischemic Heart Disease, Cerebrovascular Disease, and Hypertension

It is of interest to refer briefly to the prevalence of these diseases in the first round of the community health survey of Kiryat Yovel in 1969 to 1971 (Table 7-4). In the adult population of some 5000 men

TABLE 7-4

The Prevalence Rates* of Ischemic Heart Disease, Cerebrovascular Accidents, and Hypertension in Men and Women of Kiryat Yovel, 1969–1971

	AGE					
	25–34	35–44	45–54	55–64	65–74	75+
Ischemic heart disease						
Men	2.4	3.4	5.9	12.6	20.3	23.4
Women	2.1	2.1	4.1	8.4	12.5	24.2
Cerebrovascular accident						
Men	0.2	0.5	0.3	3.4	2.5	6.4
Women	0	0.4	0.5	1.0	2.5	7.7
Hypertension						
Men	4.0	11.4	19.8	32.5	38.3	49.9
Women	1.6	9.5	19.9	34.1	51.0	66.7

* Percent.

and women, hypertension (systolic BP 160 mm/Hg and over, and/or diastolic BP 95 mm/Hg and over) was common in the men and even more so in the women, especially from age 35 years onward. The prevalence rate in women rose from 20 percent in the age group 45 to 54, to more than 50 percent in those over 65, whereas in the men the corresponding prevalence was 20 to some 40 percent.

The diagnosis of ischemic heart disease was based on electrocardiographic findings and that of cerebrovascular accidents on documented hospital medical records.[12] The prevalence of ischemic heart disease in men increased from 6 percent in the age group 45 to 54 years to over 20 percent in those aged 65 to 74 years. The corresponding rates for women were 4 to 13 percent.

There was little difference in the prevalence rate of cerebrovascular disease in men and women, and the differences were not consistent at different ages. As expected, the prevalence rates are relatively low when compared with hypertension and ischemic heart disease.

THE ACTION PROGRAM

The family practice was organized to facilitate focusing attention on the development of the CHAD program for all men and women, 25 years and over, living in the practice area. There are two settings in which they have contact with their family physicians and nurses. One of these is within the regular primary care framework of the practice, at the health center or at home, when the opportunity may be taken to focus on any aspect of the CHAD program. The other setting is the special CHAD clinic organized for the purpose.

Throughout, it must be borne in mind that we have a double objective in respect to each risk factor. These are related but nevertheless different specific objectives, the one related to the individual patient and the other to the community as a whole. Thus, in regard to weight reduction, for the individual patient, the target was a weight below 10 percent above the standard. In the community as a whole, our aim was to shift the curve of distribution of relative weights to the left, and in so doing reduce the prevalence of weights that were 10 percent or more above the standard.

The family physicians use two situations for carrying out the CHAD program with their patients. First, they invite patients to visit them at special times set aside for CHAD purposes. This soon developed into the "CHAD clinics" of the family practice, with each of the family physicians seeing the patients of their particular practices. Thus, while this is a special clinic, it is not carried out by visiting specialists. It is a responsibility of the primary care physicians themselves, using consultative services as they would for other cases in their practice. The second situation in which the family physicians review and supervise their patients is in the course of their daily contacts with patients seeking their care. For example, a patient attending with a mild complaint might be checked to see if all CHAD program requirements are being met, and further appointments made if necessary.

The CHAD Clinics

As indicated in the review of the CHAD health team, both physicians and nurses conduct CHAD clinics together and separately. These clinics were started in June 1971 as physician clinics, but by June 1972 special nurse CHAD clinics were initiated. These special sessions are usually held in the late afternoons and early evenings, and individuals or several family members are invited to attend. At the initial session, the findings are explained and discussed. The recommended care program, prepared by the CHAD team, is then outlined, with special emphasis on prevention and what needs to be done in order to comply with the program. Individuals may need further assessment or investigation, modification of diet, advice on cigarette smoking or physical exercise, and input on the importance of keeping appointments with the nurse or doctor and adhering to medication advice.

The Family Physician's Role. Physicians have clinical, epidemiologic, and administrative functions in this program. The senior family physicians have been involved in the planning and execution of CHAD since its initiation. In the early stages of the program, each case was reviewed in detail by the CHAD team as a whole, but more recently these reviews have been carried out by the family physicians in discussion with the nurses. The physician conducts the initial examination and assessment of health status; decisions are made on the action program in consultation with the individual or family. Subsequently, they see all cases referred by the nurses, and also make periodic progress assessment of their patients with heart and cerebrovascular disease, diabetes, and other CHAD conditions. They also meet with the nurses to review progress of the CHAD program in respect of all adults in the community. The tendency in such a program is to neglect those who have no risk factors, the so-called normals, and thereby fail to initiate primary preventive measures for this group.

Periodic epidemiologic reviews of different aspects of CHAD are prepared by the family physicians, working together with the health recorder/statistician of the team and epidemiologists of the department of social medicine. Increasingly, these reviews are focusing on evaluation of the program.

More recently, the physicians have been actively engaged in discussions of this program with members of the community and other agencies in the area. This is leading toward more active participation of the community in the CHAD program itself, and especially extension of special aspects of it to other neighborhoods of the area.

The Family Nurse's Role.   In the CHAD clinics this involves two main functions:

1. Participation in the physician's CHAD clinics, receiving patients, making progress notes, carrying out routine procedures such as weighing, measuring blood pressure, and participating in the discussions on the CHAD care program with the physician and members of her families.
2. At her own CHAD session, functioning as a relatively independent nurse practitioner, she follows through the routines of the program, checking blood pressures and weight, taking blood specimens and doing electrocardiograms, conducting dietary interviews, and discussing any questions the individual wishes, such as weight reduction, stopping cigarette smoking, side effects of medication, or more personal problems.

All this requires interviewing and counseling skills, as well as health education and judgment as to the need for referral to the family physician. Each family nurse cares for her own CHAD patients, thus ensuring the integration of this community program into her practice, in much the same way as for other community-oriented programs, such as the promotion of growth and development of infants and young children.

For these various purposes, each nurse maintains a special family nurse register in the form of a compact notebook, with separate sections for each of the community programs. This record includes lists of the names and addresses of all those in the program, their health conditions, special treatments, and future appointments.

The two physicians and four nurses of the family practice together conducted 176 special CHAD sessions during the course of 1978. The nurses averaged 24 separate sessions each, 95 in all, and the physicians conducted 81 sessions. The average attendance at each nurse session was 5.4, and at the physician sessions 5.8.

The initiation of intervention follows review of a patient's risk status, together with the preparation of a special health maintenance plan to meet the needs of each individual. Basically, the intervention involves consideration of diet, physical exercise, cigarette smoking, and medication. The individuals are classified into several care categories depending on their health condition and risk status. There are (1) those that need long-term medication, advice on behavior, and frequent checks of their condition; (2) those also with risk factors requiring counseling and less intensive surveillance; and (3) those in whom no risk factors have as yet been found, but who need health counseling and periodic but less frequent assessment.

Of the 729 persons in the CHAD program of the family practice, in 1978, 34 percent were in the first category, 51 percent in the second, and only 15 percent in the third. The present aim is for the physician or nurse to have planned appointments with the treatment group three times annually, the special counseling and surveillance group twice, and the third group at least once a year.

Eligibility for Initiation
and Continuation of Program

As indicated earlier, there were 956 candidates eligible for admission into the CHAD program; the eligibility was based on three main criteria, namely, they lived in a defined area of Kiryat Yovel, which was a part of the health center's family practice, were aged 25 or over, and had been examined in the community health survey (1969–1971). Of these, 782 were initiated into the program between 1971 and 1973. By February 1979, 531 were still in the program, 159 had left the area, 75 had died, and 17 had dropped out. Thus, 10 years from the beginning of the community health survey, 68 percent of those originally included remained in the CHAD program.

Five years after the first community health survey, a second round of examinations of all who were in the program and new candidates for admission was carried out. The new persons were those who lived in the defined area and had reached the age of 25 years since the first round of examinations, as well as new arrivals in the area. Of the 287 new persons examined, 194 (68 percent) were initiated into the CHAD program in 1977. Over one-fifth of these new arrivals in the area had left it between the time of their examination in the second round of the community health study, 1975–1976, and the period of initiation into the CHAD program, 1977. The high mobility through the defined area is an important consideration in conducting and evaluating such a program. In all, there were 725 persons in the program at that time, made up of 531 who were of the first group initiated and the 194 of the second group.

In the light of the first 10 years of experience, especially with the mobility of the population, discussions are now under way to modify the procedure of incorporating new candidates for CHAD. It is felt that periodic 5-year examinations of all those already in the program are satisfactory for review purposes and evaluation of the program. However, age cohorts attaining the age of 25 years should be examined as they become eligible. This should apply both to established residents and new arrivals, aged 25 years and over. Thus, it is proposed to separate such initial examinations from the periodic 5-year reviews, for evaluation of progress of those in the program.

Another proposal now under consideration is the possibility of extending the program to younger age groups. This will be a junior CHAD project.

Program Outlines

The program outlines have been prepared and are updated for each element of the overall program. The hub of this multifactorial program is the emphasis on diet and nutrition, supported by other important aspects of intervention. While the action is epidemiologically based and focused on the adult community as a whole, it is adapted to the specific needs of each individual. It includes health examinations; advice regarding diet, exercise, or smoking; and medicinal treatment of conditions such as high blood pressure, diabetes, or hypercholesterolemia. It depends on careful attention to individual diagnosis and treatment, which is a function of the special CHAD clinics, as well as ongoing surveillance and evaluation of the program for the community as a whole, not only for those under treatment.

Diet and Nutrition

A sample of 200 individuals had a detailed dietary interview at home by a nutritionist. The dietary survey findings associated with the high rate of obesity in adults indicated that the following modifications were necessary:

1. Reduction in calories, with special emphasis on sugar and sugar-sweetened foods.
2. Reduction of high-saturated fats, especially foods commonly eaten in this community, sour cream, hard margarine, butter, and fat cheeses, and their replacement by foods with low saturated-fat content, such as low fat content milk preparations, poultry, and fish. Use of the readily available unsaturated fatty acid cooking oils was encouraged.
3. Reduction of the high egg consumption.

Diet is discussed with all adults in the program, especially those who are overweight and those with high serum cholesterol levels or diabetes mellitus. Suitable methods of nutrition education in a family practice need much attention. It is an extremely important area, in need of change, yet for many reasons it is not readily modified. Diet surveys are time-consuming, expensive, and not very reliable. It is especially difficult to effect change in the dietary habits of people who feel well, when their habits reflect the customs of the society in which they live. The values attached to certain foods, such as milk and eggs in Israel, cannot readily be questioned when so much effort has been invested in successfully building an agricultural foundation and cooperative distribution enterprises, in which these products have figured so importantly. A national program aiming to change values and customary practices of the society could be supported by health education and counseling in primary health services. This is not to suggest that a primary care practice should wait until the society as a whole is the focus of attention; rather it should make more effective use of primary health care as an instrument promoting health through more intensive nutrition education.

Cigarette Smoking

The role of cigarette smoking as an independent risk factor for ischemic heart disease has been well established for some years. The first steps taken by our department were to discourage doctors and nurses from smoking, with considerable success, especially among the doctors. Those who do continue to smoke have been requested not to smoke in the health center building, especially in clinics, offices, and all places used by the public. With regard to the community, the objective is to advise smokers to stop doing so and to discourage young people from acquiring the habit. This is done at CHAD sessions with individuals and families, and with all patients attending for care. There are also notices requesting no smoking in the health center building and wall posters illustrating the harmful effects of smoking.

The aims are to decrease the proportion of smokers in the community and, at the same time, to decrease the mean number of cigarettes smoked by those who persist.

Hypertension and Blood Pressure

The diet and nutrition program outlined above has much relevance to this risk factor. Not only has the aim been to reduce the prevalence of overweight, but in addition, reduction of salt intake has been encouraged.

The aim of antihypertensive treatment and behavior change was to reduce the blood pressure to levels below 160/95, and if possible, below 140/90. The objective for the community as a whole was to shift the blood pressure distribution curve to the left, that is, in the direction of lower values, with special emphasis on reduction of the prevalence of hypertension.

Serum Cholesterol Level

All persons were advised to use a cholesterol-lowering diet with special emphasis on those with higher risk levels above 240 mg/100 ml, and the borderline risk group, 200–239 mg. Medication, clofibrate, was used until recently for all cases with an initial serum cholesterol level exceeding 300 mg/100 ml, and for those above 240 mg/100 ml whose levels did not drop in response to dietary treatment. With the recent report of the possible side effects of this drug, its use has been reduced.[13,14] The objective was to reduce the prevalence of high and borderline risk serum cholesterol levels, and at the same time to modify the distribution of serum cholesterol levels in the community as a whole toward lower values.

Diabetes

The treatment for diabetes has been diet control and, where necessary, insulin or the oral medications. These last drugs have been used much less since the controversy as to their safety.

Apart from treatment for diabetes itself, careful surveillance and active intervention are focused on the cardiovascular status. This is of considerable importance in such a program, since diabetes is common in this community (Table 7-1) and there is a high risk for cardiovascular disease in those who have diabetes in such communities.

SURVEILLANCE AND
PERIODIC REVIEWS

In a community program such as this, conducted through primary health care, it is essential to check whether we are doing what we set out to do in carrying out different aspects of the program, and to check the effect on the practice itself and on the health status of the community. The record system includes a key record, the surveillance card register, which is maintained by the nurse coordinator of the program. It records details of the various procedures according to the dates they are due to be done. Appointments are made, and the required procedures checked when completed. Thus, this card is the key for the CHAD clinics. When the patient comes in response to the invitation, the nurse reviews the different aspects of the program, carries out any investigations or treatments required, and if necessary refers the patient to the physician. Every effort is made to contact those who do not respond, especially the healthy younger persons who are asymptomatic and do not feel the need for care.

In addition to the surveillance record, several other individual progress records are maintained in the individual's clinical file, as well as medication cards indicating the nature of the drug, its dose and frequency, and date of issue. The records are kept in the pharmacy.

Surveillance of health and its determinants and of compliance with the program, both by the health team and the population, is an ongoing process, which is reviewed periodically at special weekly community medicine reviews. All members of the professional staff of the department of social medicine and the health center attend these weekly sessions, which are also used as teaching sessions in the graduate curriculum of studies. These sessions, which have been described more fully in Chapter 4, are an important stimulus in the carrying out of programs. Presenting aspects of the work being done by a health team, in respect of a community medicine program for which it has responsibility in a primary care practice, is a considerable demand on the staff concerned, but is nevertheless a very worthwhile investment. Comment by one's peers, engaged in similar epidemiologically oriented community programs but focused on different health problems, is an important stimulus and support for further endeavor.

EVALUATION OF
THE CHAD PROGRAM

The elements of the program that will be evaluated are:

1. The integration of this community medicine program in primary health care, that is, in the general family practice of the departmental health center.
2. The knowledge that a community health survey contributes to a family practice.
3. The extent to which the program is carried out.
4. Changes in the distribution and prevalence of risk factors, namely, cigarette smoking, blood pressure, serum cholesterol, relative weight.

The Integration of CHAD as a Community
Medicine Program in the Primary
Health Care of the Family Practice

Long-term programs for the control of diseases of the circulatory system are now being subjected to trial in a number of studies. Although there is general agreement that there is a strong case for well-controlled trials, opinion is divided on the justification for widespread screening procedures and referral for treatment of the cases found. Some want more evidence of patient compliance and effectiveness before such measures are advocated.[15] Others, feeling the urgency of health problems such as hypertension, emphasize the necessity for more attention to its recognition and treatment.[16-20] While a number of programs with encouraging results continue to be reported,[21,22] there is need for a special organizational framework.[23]

A major objective of this CHAD program has been to test the hypothesis that a primary health care setting is well suited for the development of such a community medicine trial, involving both primary and secondary prevention of a community syndrome, which is of major public health importance in the country. The trial, therefore, involved two major tasks: first, to establish a special health team composed mainly of members of the family practice team itself; and second, to define a control population, which would be examined and followed through for purposes of comparing the outcome of the family practice CHAD program with the control.

The training of staff and the development of a well-functioning health team in the family practice has been steadily achieved. Evidence for this statement is as follows:

Direction of the Program.   The original direction of the program was the responsibility of non-family physicians, namely, the head of the department and a senior colleague, who functioned as epidemiologists and administrators. The senior family physicians worked with them and had the responsibility of guiding the decisions in relation to their feasibility in the practice. One of them is now director of the CHAD program, functioning as epidemiologist and clinician and using the resources of the department of social medicine for consultation in planning, surveillance, and evaluation. The other senior family physician, who is now in charge of the health center, is also actively involved in the program and participates in all decisions involving modifications.

The Nursing Program.   There is a special nurse coordinator of this program. This is so for all the community medicine programs we have now developed within the framework of the primary care of the health center. She has been responsible for this function since the inception of the program and has successfully involved all the senior family nurses in the practice. Whereas this nurse coordinator initially took almost all the nursing responsibility, each family nurse is now, and has been for a number of years, responsible for the CHAD program in families of her area, including conduct of a CHAD clinic and participation with the family physicians in their special CHAD sessions when these involve members of her families.

Records and Statistical Analysis.   The chief recorder of the health center, a statistician trained in public health, has been a member of the team since its inception and has played an increasingly important decision-making role. She is also a member of the departmental epidemiology and biostatistics unit, and is thus able to use this unit as a referral resource.

Community Organization and Health Education.   The community organizer on the health center staff is a member of the CHAD team and is involved in furthering its objectives through his links with formal and informal groups of Kiryat Yovel communities, as well as of Jerusalem as a whole. The most recent development has been the formation of an overall community group, involving staff of the health center, other agencies active in Kiryat Yovel, and most important, members of the community itself. The CHAD program has been discussed in this group, and other medical clinics in the area are now planning some development along these lines.

Thus, the CHAD program is now as well integrated into the family practice as is the older maternal and child health care service. Both are combined curative and preventive care programs, carried out by the family practice team members themselves, within frameworks specially defined to ensure that both community and individual orientations receive the attention they need, if community-oriented primary health care is to be an ongoing established feature of this teaching health center.

The Contribution of a Community
Health Survey to a Family Practice

Using a primary care setting for the development of community medicine requires epidemiologic method in the development of knowledge about the community's health. While some of this knowledge accumulates in the course of daily practice attending to the needs of patients, there are large segments of the population registered with the practice who do not use it unless they feel ill. That this is true even in a teaching health center is evidenced by the findings arising from the community health survey that was conducted before CHAD was initiated.

One of the most interesting results of this early experience was the number of new cases found by the community health survey of the "family practice" population, compared with the percentage previously known (Table 7-5).[24] Among the more important findings were

TABLE 7-5

Findings in Men and Women of a Family Practice Before
and after a Community Health Survey (CHS)

	MEN			WOMEN		
	25-44	45-64	65 +	25-44	45-64	65 +
Blood pressure						
% *not* taken before CHS	48	11	18	23	13	14
% diastolic BP 90 mm Hg or over:						
known before CHS	14	51	62	16	67	75
after CHS	37	66	74	28	76	80
Serum cholesterol level						
% *not* taken before CHS	75	41	36	72	36	37
% with level 240 mg/ 100 ml +:						
known before CHS	1	31	31	7	44	49
after CHS	7	42	33	13	49	61

the expected differences in frequency of blood pressure and serum cholesterol examinations between the younger men and women (25 to 44 years). The higher attendance of women generally, especially for prenatal and postnatal care, with their babies and younger children, increased the likelihood of their blood pressures being measured. This fact, together with the survey findings of a high prevalence of hypertension and borderline high blood pressure, of hypercholesterolemia, diabetes mellitus, and overweight, demonstrates the need for preventive clinical services for men, whether in the neighborhood where they live or at work. Such services are needed for all age groups of men, among whom there is a steep rise with age in most of the above risk factors.

A Measurement of the Extent to Which the Team Was Carrying Out the Program, and the Response of the Community

Periodic reviews of this important subject are made and presented at the weekly community medicine rounds of the department of social medicine and its health center in Kiryat Yovel. As indicated earlier, the adult population eligible for CHAD is classified into three categories: (1) those in need of medication; (2) those in need of special counseling and surveillance; and (3) those with no risk factors found on examination, as well as cigarette smokers with no other risk factors. The aims and achievements for 1978 are summarized in the following data:

	Category		
	1	*2*	*3*
Number of persons in category	250	373	106
Percentage having at least one contact (1978)	95.6	81.2	66
Number of contacts per person			
Aim for the year	3	2	1
Actual average	2.1	1.2	0.8

There is clearly a need for increase in contact with well people of Category 3, if primary prevention is to be a more important feature of this program and if we are to make greater impact on cigarette smokers of this predominantly younger age group of adults.

Changes in the Distribution and
Prevalence of Some Risk Factors

A preliminary evaluation of the effectiveness of the CHAD program has been reported.[25] As this program is the first trial of its kind in Israel, and differs from other multifactorial cardiovascular risk factor trials in that it is developed within the framework of a primary care family practice, we designed it as a controlled evaluative study with the following features:

The evaluation of effectiveness was to be based on changes in the prevalence of risk factors in the population involved in the CHAD program, compared with those of the control adult population, aged 25 years and over, living in adjacent areas of Kiryat Yovel.

The data were obtained from two community health surveys, the initial in 1969 to 1971 and the next in 1975 to 1976, using standardized methods.

The information used for this preliminary analysis presents the findings among men 35 years and over who were examined in both surveys. Apart from their involvement in both surveys, the men of the control population were not exposed to the CHAD program, but the findings of the surveys were sent to their doctors. In this analysis, there were 211 men in the CHAD population and 709 in the control population. The CHAD group were older and had a lower standard of education and a lower social class distribution. A much higher proportion were of North African origin (40 percent vs. 11 percent), and a much lower proportion were born in Israel (7 percent vs. 26 percent) or in Europe or America (29 percent vs. 47 percent). There was also a lower proportion of older settlers in the CHAD population (11 percent vs. 37 percent).

Because of the disparity in ages, comparisons between the two population groups are based on age-standardized distribution where relevant. The succeeding parts of the present evaluation are based on the report published by Abramson et al.[25]

Changes in Behavior. *Cigarette Smoking.*   In both groups, there was a decline in the number of smokers between the 1970 and 1975 surveys, more marked in the family practice population than in the control group. This is indicated by the following facts:

	Population of the Family Practice (CHAD)			Control Population		
	1970	*1975*	*Change*	*1970*	*1975*	*Change*
Age-standardized percentage of smokers	54.4	41.5	-12.9	44.6	38.4	-6.2

In the family practice population, there were 32 smokers who became nonsmokers, and three former nonsmokers who started smoking, an odds ratio of 10.7 : 1. The corresponding figures in the control population were 76 and 29, an odds ratio of 2.6 : 1. When the smoking habits were compared after taking account of the differences in age, as well as in the number of cigarettes smoked in 1970 and then of the number smoked in 1975, the difference between the two populations was significant.

The main change was due to a decrease of light smokers, there being little change in the proportions of those who smoked 20 or more cigarettes daily.

Physical Activity.   Self-appraisal of physical activity, using a scale from 1 (least active) to 5 (most active), showed no significant differences between the two populations, and there was little difference between the findings of the 1970 and 1975 surveys.

Diet.   In the 1975 survey, 37 percent of men in the family practice population (CHAD), compared with 23 percent in the control population, reported that they kept to a diet for one or more of the following reasons: weight control, cholesterol level, blood pressure, or heart disease. This considerable difference is significant. The differences between the two populations were also significant in respect to the various reasons for dieting. Thus, when we controlled for age, 28.5 percent of the family practice population stated they were on a diet to control or reduce weight, compared with 20.5 percent in the control group. There were also 6.1 percent of the men in the CHAD population who were controlling their diet for reasons connected with cholesterol, compared with the corresponding proportion of 1.4 percent in the control population.

Blood Pressure Change.   The change in the blood pressure in the family practice population has been compared with the control in respect of (1) the prevalence of hypertension in both community health surveys; and (2) the means and frequency distributions of systolic and diastolic blood pressure in the two populations.

The Prevalence of Hypertension.   With the cutting points of 160 mm Hg or over for systolic blood pressure, and/or 95 mm Hg or over for diastolic blood presure as the definition of hypertension, the data in Table 7–6 summarize the differences between the two populations of men aged 35 years and over.

While hypertension declined in both populations, that of the family practice in which the CHAD program was carried out did so to a greater extent.

TABLE 7-6

Changes in the Prevalence of Hypertension in Men in the
Family Practice (CHAD) and Control Populations

	FAMILY PRACTICE		CONTROL	
	1970	1975	1970	1975
Age-standardized prevalence rate of hypertension	24.1%	14.5%	20.4%	16.0%
Change between 1970 and 1975		-9.6%		-4.3%
Number of men who changed categories between 1970 and 1975				
Moved out of hypertension category (a)		35		80
Moved into hypertension category (b)		13		49
Odds ratio a : b*		2.7		1.6
p		0.001		0.004
Difference between the two populations in their odds ratios, controlling for age		1.7		
p		0.094		

*Odds ratio a : b expresses tendency to move out of hypertension category.

A striking finding in regard to high systolic blood pressures in the CHAD population was the considerably lower age-standardized prevalence in 1975 than in 1970. At 160 mm Hg the decrease was by one-third and at 170 mm Hg it was by one-half. This is in marked contrast to the control group in which there was relatively little change. While both groups showed a decline in age-standardized high diastolic blood pressure (95 mm Hg and over), the CHAD group declined by 10.2 percent (from 17.4 to 7.2 percent) and the control population by 6.1 percent (from 15.8 to 9.7 percent).[25]

The Mean Blood Pressure and Frequency Distribution of Systolic and Diastolic Blood Pressure. The mean systolic and diastolic blood pressures of the men in the CHAD population declined by 4.4 mm Hg over the 5-year period, compared with a decrease of only 1.1 mm Hg in the control population. The decline in the mean diastolic blood pressure was also greater in the CHAD population, 4.6 mm Hg, than in the control population, 2.5 mm Hg (Table 7-7).

The differences in changes in the means of the CHAD and control group were significant, controlling for age. Comparing the frequency distributions, there was a clear shift to the lower values in the CHAD group in both systolic and diastolic blood pressure, whereas in the

TABLE 7-7

**Changes in the Mean Blood Pressure of Men in the Family
Practice (CHAD) and Control Populations**

	FAMILY PRACTICE	CONTROL POPULATION
Systolic blood pressure		
Mean in mm Hg		
1970	133.8	132.4
1975	129.4	131.3
Difference	4.4	1.1
Diastolic blood pressure		
Mean in mm Hg		
1970	83.1	82.5
1975	78.5	80.0
Difference	4.6	2.5

control population there was little change in the distribution curve for
systolic blood pressures of the men, and the shift in diastolic blood
pressure distribution was less marked than in the CHAD population.
The changes in the frequency distribution of blood pressure in the
CHAD population were especially marked at the higher levels of both
systolic (160 mm Hg and above) and diastolic (90 mm Hg and above),
whereas in the control population the slight decrease in the prevalence
of high systolic pressures was more apparent only at levels of 200 mg
Hg and over.

Serum Cholesterol.   The age-standardized prevalence rate of hypercholesterolemia (serum cholesterol level 250 mg/100 ml or over was
used) declined in both the CHAD and control populations. In the
CHAD population, it declined from 18.0 percent in the 1970 survey to
9.4 percent in 1975, and in the control group, from 22.1 to 17.0 percent. The number of cases that moved out of the high category in the
CHAD group was 25, while 10 moved into the high group, an odds
ratio of 2.5. The corresponding figures for the control population of
men was 81 and 50, an odds ratio of 1.6. This change in both populations was significant, but controlling for age, the ratio expressing the
difference between the two populations, 1.4, was not significant.

These differences in the prevalence of hypercholesterolemia are
reflected in the decline in the mean age-standardized level of serum
cholesterol in both populations. The CHAD group declined from a
mean of 212.0 mg/100 ml (S.D. 44.6) in the 1970 survey to 206 (S.D.
37.5) in 1975. Corresponding figures for the control population were
217.7 to 214.1. The difference of –6.0 mg/100 ml in the CHAD popula-

tion mean level, and of −3.6 mg/100 ml in the control group, are both significant, but the difference between the change in the two populations is not.

Weight Change.   There was no change in the mean weight of the CHAD men between 1970 and 1975, 70.5 kg (S.D. 11.5) and 70.4 kg (S.D. 11.4); there was also almost no change in the percentage classified as being overweight (20 percent or more over the standard weight), 23.3 percent in the 1970 survey and 23.6 percent in the 1975 survey. Both these sets of findings are based on age-standardized figures. The odds ratio was 1.0, with 19 men moving into the overweight category and 19 out of it. The control group differed from these findings. There was a slight but significant change upward in the age-standardized mean, i.e., 72.2 kg in 1970 and 72.5 kg in 1975, and the age-standardized prevalence rate of overweight men increased from 24.8 to 26.4 percent. There were 43 men who moved out of the high category compared with 58 who moved into this category, an odds ratio of 0.7.

The difference between the two populations in respect to their mean weight changes, CHAD −0.1 kg and control +0.3, controlling for age, was of borderline significance.

CONCLUSION

Despite the real difficulties in setting up and maintaining a community program such as CHAD in a highly mobile population, there have been encouraging changes. The first program evaluation indicates its effectiveness in several important aspects, namely, a decline in cigarette smoking, though mainly in lighter smokers; a decline in the prevalence of hypertension and in the curve of distribution of blood pressure; and a decrease in cholesterol levels. Perhaps most important has been the development of a primary health care team, willing and able to carry out an epidemiologically based community health program in their practice, together with the growing participation of the community.

The program outlined here differs from other multifactorial preventive programs in the United States[26] and Europe[27-29] in that it is being carried out within the primary health care of a family practice in a neighborhood health center. It is focused on all the adults of the family practice, and members of the health team involved are predominantly the staff of the family practice. A major objective, which has been achieved, was to gain experience in how to integrate community medicine with primary health care by the use of both epidemiologic and clinical skills. In doing this, a community-oriented primary health care practice has been established, and shown to be feasible and effective.

The approach we have used precludes some of the disadvantages of mass screening. It includes some of the best features of such screening, for example, the recognition of previously undiagnosed abnormalities, and is done by physicians or a primary health care team who know their patients. Putting the screening and its follow-through in this framework has no doubt been a major reason for the high response rate of the community. Furthermore, this approach has extended the functions of the survey from screening of cases, and hence secondary prevention, to a more epidemiologic orientation, with analysis of the frequency distribution in the community, and of risk factors and relevant behavior variables, and hence to primary prevention. Thus, the mass screening approach to case finding is modified to become a community health survey of a known population. This is accomplished in a less anonymous, more intimate setting of primary care, which focuses on both primary and secondary prevention, on the individual's well-being, and on the health status of the community as a whole.

In a program such as CHAD, much time and effort are needed for developing a system of primary care practice which includes community diagnosis, intervention, surveillance, and evaluation. The more common and the more serious the community health implications, the more justifiable it is to make such an investment. Active intervention demands even more. If a family practice or other forms of primary care are to be used as a major instrument in community medicine, that is, to change the state of health of the community and not only of a particular individual, there must be evidence that such action is likely to be effective. Hence the need for evaluation of program trials aimed toward effecting a change in health care in the community.

REFERENCES

1. Kark SL: Epidemiology and Community Medicine. New York, Appleton, 1974, p 430
2. Epstein FH, Ostrander LD Jr, Johnson BC, et al.: Epidemiological studies of cardiovascular disease in a total community: Tecumseh, Michigan. Ann Intern Med 62:1170, 1965
3. Epstein FH, Francis T, Hayner NS, et al.: Prevalence of chronic diseases and distribution of selected physiologic variables in a total community, Tecumseh, Michigan. Am J Epidemiol 81:307, 1965

4. Epstein FH: Hyperglycemia. A risk factor in coronary artery disease. Circulation 36:609, 1967

5. Keen H, Rose G, Pyke DA, et al.: Blood sugar and arterial disease. Lancet 2:505, 1965

6. Kannel WB, McGee DL: Diabetes and cardiovascular disease. The Framingham study. JAMA 241:2035, 1979

7. Peritz E, Dreyfus F, Halevi HS, et al.: Mortality of Adult Jews in Israel 1950–1967. Special Series No. 409. Jerusalem, Central Bureau of Statistics, 1973

8. Statistical Abstract of Israel No. 29. Jerusalem, Central Bureau of Statistics, 1978

9. Abramson JH, Kark SL, Epstein LM, et al.: A community health study in Jerusalem. Aims, design, response. Isr J Med Sci 15:725, 1979

10. Kark SL, Kark E, Hopp C, et al.: The control of hypertension, atherosclerotic diseases, and diabetes in a family practice. J R Coll Gen Pract 26:157, 1976

11. Interdepartmental Committee on Nutrition for National Defense: Manual for Nutrition Surveys, 2nd ed. Bethesda, Maryland, U.S. National Institutes of Health, 1963, chap 9

12. Kark SL, Gofin J, Abramson JH, et al.: The prevalence of selected health characteristics of men. A community health survey in Jerusalem. Isr J Med Sci 15:732, 1979

13. Committee of Principal Investigators: A cooperative trial in the primary prevention of ischaemic heart disease using clofibrate. Br Heart J 40:1069, 1978

14. Oliver MF: Cholesterol, coronaries, clofibrate and death. N Engl J Med 299:1360, 1978

15. Sackett DL: Screening for disease. Cardiovascular disease. Lancet 2:1189, 1974

16. Coope J: A screening clinic for hypertension in general practice. J R Coll Gen Pract 24:161, 1974

17. Stamler J: Acute myocardial infarction—progress in primary prevention. Br Heart J 33 (Suppl) 145, 1971

18. Hart JT: The management of high blood pressure in general practice. J R Coll Gen Pract 25:160, 1975

19. Wilber JA: Hypertension as a community problem. Prev Med 3:353, 1974

20. Abramson, JH, Hopp C: The control of cardiovascular disease factors in the elderly. Prev Med 5:32, 1976

21. Rudnick KV, Sackett DL, Hirst S, et al.: Hypertension in a family practice. Can Med Assoc J 117:492, 1977

22. Alderman MH, Schoenbaum EE: Detection and treatment of hypertension at the work site. N Engl J Med 293:65, 1975

23. Engelland AL, Alderman MH, Powell HB: Blood pressure control in private practice: A case report. Am J Public Health 69:25, 1979

24. Abramson JH, Epstein LM, Kark SL, et al.: The contribution of a health survey to a family practice. Scand J Soc Med 1:33, 1973

25. Abramson JH, Hopp C, Gofin J, et al.: A community program for the control of cardiovascular risk factors. J Community Health 4:3, 1979

26. The Multiple Risk Factor Intervention Trial (MRFIT): A national study of primary prevention of coronary heart disease. JAMA 235:825, 1976

27. World Health Organization European Collaborative Group: An international control trial in the multifactorial prevention of coronary heart disease. Int J Epidemiol 3:219, 1974
28. Report of a WHO Working Group: The prevention of coronary heart disease. Copenhagen, WHO Regional Office for Europe, 1977
29. Koskela K, Puska P, Tuomilehto J: The North Karelia Project: A first evaluation. Int J Health Educ 19:59, 1976

CHAPTER 8

COMMUNITY HEALTH CARE IN A RURAL AFRICAN POPULATION

Of what relevance is this chapter, in which we look back 40 years to our experience in initiating community-oriented primary health care in a peasant community? We believe that the approach we and our African colleagues were able to develop has relevance to the present day for such communities. Even more, perhaps, the experience we had in changing our own basic medical orientation, and in training the new types of community health workers needed for such services, may be of interest to the many who are spearheading a worldwide quest for improved health care of communities, families, and individuals.

Most of the world's population still live in rural areas. Peasant communities constitute the greatest part of the population in many developing countries. Their human skills and technologic resources are poorly developed, and even in those countries in which they predominate in numbers, the health system barely reaches out to them. Unfortunately, in many developing countries, the main features of the health system have been modeled on that of more developed countries, with concentration on the building of relatively large, well-equipped hospitals in the cities. Some relate this policy of governments to politicians' need for visible signs of achievement. The 1000-bed hospital is far more striking evidence of progress than the development of many community health centers or clinics scattered through the rural communities. It is our feeling that this is true of more advanced countries as well. Even in cities, the development of community-based services is apparently less rewarding for the politician, the president of a voluntary organization, and even the health service administrator. While tribute is often paid to those pioneers

Dr. Emily Kark is co-author of this chapter.

who establish community-based services in deprived communities, when financial constraints press upon a government or voluntary organizations, it is the rural community health programs or inner-city community health projects that are curtailed or even abolished.

The fact is that impoverished peasant communities, together with their other difficulties and privations, are deprived of the most elementary forms of modern health care. There have been many projects in rural community health care, from each of which there has been much to learn, but it is only in recent years that health care especially appropriate for rural peasant communities has become part of the social policy of government. There is a widening appreciation of the role which community health has in community development, and hence the determination of some governments to change the state of health by using innovative approaches involving fresh orientations and new types of community health workers. This has been reviewed in Chapter 1 of this volume. The World Health Organization's sponsorship of the drive toward appropriate forms of primary care is perhaps the most encouraging sign for the future.[1-4]

It was in such a peasant community that the Polela Health Center was established in 1940 as a pilot project in rural community health services. Looking back on that early experience, we are struck by the resemblance of the social and health problems of the Polela community with those of other deprived rural communties we have since observed in other countries. While every community has its unique characteristics, related to its history, culture, and habitat, the similarities between peasant communities extend through their social, economic, agricultural, educational, and health status. Poverty, malnutrition, and disease are common dominating features of community living. Polela was a very poor rural community.

Polela is situated in the foothills of the Drakensberg mountain range, which at this point separates Kwa-Zulu of South Africa from LeSotho. Here several Zulu tribal communities lived a life of poverty, with all its implications for disease and malnutrition. Their homesteads were clusters of huts, made of wattle and daub with thatched roofs, spread along the mountain slopes, with fast-flowing rivers cutting deep valleys below. They were exposed to heavy summer rainstorms and freezing winters, and communication was limited to walking and horse riding.

The people who now live there arrived following the southern migration of whole tribes in the face of defeat in the Zulu wars of the nineteenth century. It began when Tshaka, a Zulu chief, was building the Zulu nation by military conquest and subjugation of the tribes living in what is now Kwa-Zulu. The tribe in whose area our health center was established were descendants of these people who, together with others, left their homes farther north, eventually settling in the area of Polela. Older men and women with whom we spoke of earlier times when they were children, remembered numbers of families still arriving to settle the mountain slopes where their children and grandchildren now live. Our estimate was that this final migration took place in the later years of the nineteenth century. They were a pastoral people rather than a settled agricultural peasantry, a fact that helps to explain the devastation that had been wrought by soil erosion in this beautiful mountainous locality. The fast-flowing rivers are brown with the soil washed down from the mountainous slopes by the heavy summer rainstorms. Deep gullies cut through the fields, the rushing waters taking all before them on their way to the rivers.

The main fields were planted with maize and sorghum, the yield being insufficient to meet the basic caloric needs of the vast majority of families. Our studies indicated that most homes were buying their meager supplies of maize within 3 months of reaping their own crops. The agricultural authorities reported serious overstocking of cattle and goats, and yet our data showed that most families had limited numbers of these animals, with marked deficiencies of meat and milk in the diet. This was an indication of overpopulation. Thus, in one locality in which there were 130 homes with 887 people when we first conducted a family health census, 16 years later there were 184 homes with 1509 people, a population increase of 70 percent, or 4.4 percent per year, and an increase in the average number of persons per homestead from 6.8 to 8.2.[5] This was related to a continuing high birth rate, over 40 per 1000 population, and a considerable decline in mortality rate, an indication of the need of family planning for which the people were not yet ready.

To meet their survival needs and stave off famine, the people of Polela did what other rural communities in southern Africa were doing. Boys in their teens and men, young and middle-aged, went to the cities for all types of unskilled and semiskilled work. Their absence from home for long periods was perhaps the single most striking feature of the social structure, with profound implications for all facets of daily living and health. When the health center was initiated, this was already a well-established practice.

THE INITIATION OF THE HEALTH CENTER

The health team of the Polela Health Center evolved over a number of years, during which we were exploring ways of developing community health care in this rural area. While our experience in this center began many years ago and has been described in a number of publications,[6-17] there are aspects of its health care team that are appropriate and relevant to our present discussion.

The initial professional staff consisted of two doctors (husband and wife), one medical aide and a nurse (husband and wife), and five health assistants. All except the doctors were Zulu, and all had previous experience in health work or medical care among Africans. The doctors were young physicians, with several years of postgraduate training as interns and residents in hospital medicine, pediatrics, and surgery. One had subsequent experience in a national nutrition survey, and then in venereal disease, leprosy, and tuberculosis; the other was experienced in casualty and emergency-room care in several hospitals with African patients. The medical aide had graduated from a special 5-year course of training at university level and had several years of hospital clinical clerkships. This training followed a number of years as an assistant to a physician in charge of a mission hospital treating African patients. The nurse was a recent graduate qualified in general nursing and midwifery.

The five health assistants, all men, were the first appointees to these newly created posts. Four of them had been transferred from malaria services in which they had been field workers in other parts of the country, and one had been on the nutrition survey team mentioned above. They were trained at Polela as community health workers, whose functions included epidemography, health education, and community organization.

Activities during the first year included setting up of a general curative clinic, open to any patient; health surveys of children at school, followed by the initiation of school health services; meetings with the local doctor, magistrate, various missionaries, schoolteachers, and chiefs and elders of the various tribes; and home visits to introduce the people to our service. Information of health relevance was sought from official records, various officials, and individuals of the community. We were also called on to control epidemics of acute communicable diseases, typhus, typhoid, and smallpox.

The siting of the health center was a fortuitous decision. Located in an area populated by one of the main tribal groups of Polela, it soon became a center of various activities, especially following the establishment of the tribal chief's home and the opening of a general store, both near the health center.

At the time the health center was initiated, there was one general physician in Polela, who conducted a large private practice and also had functions as district health officer for the population of some 30,000. The nearest hospital was 40 miles away. The greatest part of medical care was provided by traditional practitioners of several kinds. These included the traditional doctor, or *inyanga*, and the diviner (diagnostician), or *isangoma*. Many of these practitioners were specialists, known by the people to have special skills in the treatment of particular disorders. There were no organized preventive services concerned with maternal and child health, health of the schoolchild, or any other defined groups in the population.

There was no information available on births and deaths, nor was there any source for data on health state or illnesses other than reports on epidemics, such as smallpox and typhoid fever, and on a limited number of cases with notifiable diseases, such as leprosy and tuberculosis. There were estimates of the population, based on incomplete census data. Maps of the district did not show the homes, and as expected there was no system of household addresses, with the result that even the limited information available on illnesses was not linked to particular households or families.

It soon became clear that if we were to plan for more effective community health care, it was necessary to develop methods for studying the state of health of the community, its health-relevant behavior, the people's varied perceptions of health and disease, the attitudes they had toward members of our health team, and their expectations of us. This led to the need for data on the community, such as its demographic, family, and social characteristics and its agricultural and other economic activities.

We also needed to train ourselves in various areas that would be essential for this work. The doctors, medical aide, and nurse had more knowledge of the basic sciences of medicine, public health, clinical work, and survey methods than did the health assistants. Thus, the medical and nursing team became the teachers of the health assistants in medical terminology, in basic medicine, and in public health subjects such as nutrition, growth and health, infectious diseases, epidemiology, and community health survey methods. The medical aide and health assistants knew more of traditional Zulu perceptions of health and disease, and of the different kinds of traditional practitioners. It took some time before the health assistants felt free enough to share their knowledge with others of the team, knowledge of a belief system they had been taught was "primitive" superstition and yet believed in sufficiently to use traditional practitioners for treatment of some of their illnesses. Sharing experience and information in these various areas of our respective expertise took much time and was the basis for mutual respect and trust between members of the health team, and for the planning of the initial health care activities and studies of the community.

THE DEFINED AREA FOR
COMMUNITY HEALTH CARE

In initiating various community health studies, we developed a working concept of an "intensive" or "defined" area. The first area defined for this purpose was named the River Valley Area (R.V.), extending over a distance of almost 10 miles along the river, which flowed through the area not far from the health center. The households were sited along the mountain slopes overlooking the river and their cultivated fields in the valley below. Defining the households of this area and allocating an address to each was an early task. There was much discussion with the people concerned, not only as to the purposes of introducing a health center address system, but also as to the use and functions of area maps, and what they considered to be a homestead. Homesteads often consisted of a number of nuclear family units, each living in separate groups of huts within a homestead of an extended or joint family. Using field compasses, we located each homestead on the map, gave it an address, and recorded the census of each family within it.

The mapping of homesteads was associated with a number of activities in the defined area: gathering of demographic information (household health census); initiating a system of recording births, deaths, and in- and out-movements; conducting surveys of health-related behavior and of the environment; and developing programs of family and community health education. These activities were carried out by the community health workers (CHW), directed and supported by the doctors and medical aide, who made regular visits to schools and homes, in addition to home calls in case of illness or during epidemics.

At the same time as these activities were taking place in the defined area, anyone attending the health center who lived in the defined area had their area addresses noted on their medical or other records. The records of members of the same family and homestead were kept together in a single family folder.

The clinical findings of various family members were compared, and were also studied in relation to the data gathered on the household during the community health surveys. Similarly, the treatment and advice given to patients at the health center were related to the health education and other actions taken by the community health workers in the course of home visits to these particular families. Initially, there were weekly team meetings, at which there was an interchange of information between the clinical workers, doctors, medical aide, and nurse, and the community health workers. Later, as the program developed, the frequency of team meetings increased. On the basis of the family diagnosis, a program of treatment and health education was planned and carried out by members of the team concerned with that family. In many cases, family consultations were held, which often involved separate sessions with the women and men of the household, or in cases concerning infants and young children, with mothers and grandmothers. One or both doctors, the medical aide, nurse, and the community health worker in whose area this family lived participated in the family consultation.

The reviews by the team were not confined to individual families. With the steady accumulation of data about the community living in the defined area, there were frequent reviews of community health problems, involving community diagnosis and decisions as to necessary action. The action included:

> Activities at the health center, in the clinic, in the health center's demonstration vegetable garden or poultry run, in special nutrition classes, or at "children's activity day" held each week. Activities in the defined area, at various homes, or in group discussions and actions, such as by a community group getting advice and help in the protection of a common water-supply point.

During the first 3 years of this approach, the defined area expanded from the original River Valley Area with its 887 people to several adjacent areas with a population of 5926. After this, the rate of expansion was slower; 15 years later the population included in the defined area was 10,500. The main factor determining the expansion was the size of the area, that is, the number of additional homes community health workers could be expected to manage, while at the same time working with the areas previously included in the program. The primary health care aspect was also an influencing factor, in that as an area of homes was included in the defined area, so people made more effective use of the clinic facilities at the health center. At first, this involved more frequent utilization of curative services, but in time, with control of much acute nutritional illness and infectious diseases, there was an increase in numbers of infants and children using the well-baby clinics and child play centers. There was also more use made by schoolchildren of the preventive and health education activities.

THE GROWTH AND FUNCTIONING
OF THE HEALTH TEAM

With the expansion of the defined area, the increased use of the health center's facilities, and the establishment of subcenters, the team also expanded. There were more doctors, medical aides, and nurses, but the most striking feature was the increased number of Polela men and women employed as community health workers, health recorders, and nurse aides, all trained by members of the health team. Their appointments to the health center team had much meaning for the Polela community. Born and raised in the area, several of them had been trained as teachers and were members of families known throughout the district. They became key members of the team, especially as community health workers.

The central or nuclear health team consisted of three groups:

Physicians and medical aides.
Nurses, midwives, and nurse aides.
Community health workers.

The main supportive team members were:

Laboratory technicians.
Health recorders.
Administrative staff.

There were no additional consultative team members at the center itself. Difficult clinical cases were taken by health center transport to the nearest hospital. We constituted our own internal referral system, for example, in team discussions of difficult cases of "possession" or other traditional syndromes of illness.

The functions of the three groups in the central team became more clearly defined as the practice developed in relation to the widening defined area. Looking back on this experience of 35 to 40 years ago, with the perception that we now have, the Polela team can be seen to have developed an integrated practice of community medicine and primary health care. Using community health care as a foundation, it extended its functions to community development as a whole. Further consideration of the roles of various members of the team is of interest, and perhaps of some importance, in the planning for community health care in the 1980s and onward. We spent much time defining the roles of each person in the team—not so much the theory, that came afterward, but on the day-to-day functioning.

In the main, functions pertaining to the clinic and personal health care were the responsibility of the doctors, medical aides, and nurses. The physicians were responsible for policy direction and administration of the health center, the main forum for decision making being the staff team meetings. The clinical work was carried out with medical aides and nurses who, in addition to their own clinical functions, acted as interpreters for the majority of doctors who came to

Polela not speaking Zulu. Extending through the greatest part of each day, these clinics involved promotive, preventive, and curative care of individuals and families. Understanding the patients and families, especially their perceptions of their illnesses, led to a dual system of diagnosis by which we were able to compare and contrast the people's concepts of illness, its causes, and its treatment in traditional terms and in terms of "modern" medicine, in which we had been trained. This allowed for an approach to health education in the clinic, and in the home and community, in which the starting point was the belief system and practice of the patient or family, and later that of the community.

Examples of Clinical Activities. Well-baby sessions included appraisal of growth and development, nutritional assessment and developmental diagnosis, with advice and treatment where necessary to grandmothers as well as mothers.

Health examinations of children and adults, with special attention to assessment of nutritional status and to common communicable diseases such as tuberculosis, syphilis, and skin diseases.

Prenatal examinations and treatment, again with focus on syphilis, other communicable diseases, and the mothers' nutritional status and diet.

Diagnosis and treatment of the sick of all ages, with certain basic routines for all patients (except when contraindicated), such as height and weight, blood pressure, blood examination for syphilis and hemoglobin level, tuberculin tests, and examination of size of thyroid (Polela was an endemic goiter region). At clinic visits, opportunity was also taken to immunize patients against important diseases in the area, such as smallpox, typhoid, and whooping cough.

Epidemiologic and Community Activities. These functions of the physicians and medical aides involved immediate responsibility for the direction of various community health programs, the planning of community health surveys, analysis of clinical and field data for community diagnosis and health surveillance, and ultimate decision on the kinds of action to be taken. They were responsible for the direction of the training and programs of work of the community health workers.

The first medical aide, because of his personal interests and the importance of the subject, became the center's specialist with regard to traditional medicine and the work of the traditional practitioners. The chief nurse was responsible for the clinic, its supervision and organization, conduct of the well-baby sessions, and general nursing treatments in the curative clinic.

Field Work.   This was carried out in the homes, in schools, or in other activities by community health workers, each having an area assignment. In addition to the functions outlined, the community health workers would often notify the clinical team of sick persons they had seen during their routine home visiting. Sometimes they brought back specimens such as sputum, urine, or feces, which led to an immediate identification of a patient as having tuberculosis or other significant illness. They were also a bridge between the clinic and the home, as in their functions of follow-up to ensure continuity of care and treatment in special cases, such as syphilis and kwashiorkor, which were initially very common conditions.

Team Leadership.   The people of Polela expected that the physicians would lead the team, as did all the staff members. The early emergence of differentiated leadership was of much interest. The medical aide, who had been a member of the founding team, was increasingly perceived as an additional leader by the people and the team, especially in important matters to the community or to its traditional mores.

The nurses developed their distinctive functions of leadership as outlined. However, at that time there was no trained nurse who could be recruited from any of the local Polela communities. Hence our qualified nursing staff in general nursing and midwifery were from other parts of the country. Several of them were married to other members of the health center staff and made their permanent homes in the area. This made an important difference in their status and acceptance by the people of Polela. By contrast, the nurse's aides appointed to the staff were young girls from homes in the area of Polela not far from the health center. Their status in the community was that of the other young girls, and their access to confidential information required that they receive careful supervision and training in the importance of maintaining confidentiality in personal and family information. As they became young adults and remained on the staff of the center, they became important contacts with the community and fulfilled a wider role than that of nurse's aides, extending into health education and acting as helpers in the growing sphere of activity of maternal and child health.

With the appointment of women from the community itself as community health workers, an increasing number of women in the community looked to these workers as leaders in community organization, especially in affairs concerning women and children.

Team Meetings.   These were an important feature of our activities. The meetings involved reviews of progress in different aspects of the work at the health center itself or in the field, exchange of information between different members of the team, and linking clinical findings and treatment with home and community findings. In this way, we aimed to ensure that all members of the team had the necessary information, with no member expected to make a breach of confidence of a patient or family. All members of the team were involved in reporting of information and in decision making. It was this kind of participation that built the health team.

ACTIVITIES OF THE HEALTH CENTER

As indicated earlier, among the first activities of the health team was the opening of a general curative clinic at the health center, which was conducted by the doctors, medical aide, and nurse, and was open to any patient from Polela itself or elsewhere.

Already, in the second year of the development of the defined area, which now included some 3000 people, 41 percent of patients seen at the central clinic of the health center came from homes in the defined area. As would be expected in a primary care service, this general clinic remained a central feature of the practice. In addition, special sessions were organized for different groups. These included maternal and infant health care, preschool child centers, school health examinations, nutritional and recreational activities for children, as well as special sessions for periodic health examinations of adults and health reviews of families.

Maternal and Child Health Care

Special sessions were arranged to ensure supervision of pregnant women, postnatal examinations, and well-child case conferences with mothers and grandmothers. Later the health center established a midwifery facility at the center itself.

Care of Infants. A considerable proportion of patients at the general curative clinic were mothers with their sick babies. The common illnesses included malnutrition, growth retardation, marasmus and kwashiorkor, acute gastroenteritis, pneumonia, and other acute illnesses, such as whooping cough and measles. Fundamental to success in care of such illnesses was having not only the means to treat and prevent them, but also to prevent recurrence.

Well-baby sessions were initially built up by referral of babies from the general clinic. The numbers of babies so referred increased steadily, and later with the inclusion of the midwifery service at the health center, babies were referred directly from there to the well-baby session. Generally, these sessions were conducted by the nursing staff of the center, who received special training for the purpose. Periodic health examinations and Gesell developmental assessments were conducted by the doctors, who also saw any mother and baby referred by the nurse.

The focus on infants was highly appreciated by the population and its leaders. Early on, over 80 percent of children under the age of 2 years in the defined area were attending the health center during the course of a year. Later, special subcenters were established 5 to 15 miles away from the center, in order to meet the increased demand for this type of service and bring it nearer to the homes of the people.

Two- to Five-Year-Olds. It was not long before the needs of preschool children of this age group were defined. Again we were much concerned with malnutrition and preventable or readily treatable communicable diseases. A special play group was organized at the health center by the first woman community health worker we had appointed.

Its success was followed by the establishment of a number of other such play groups in various parts of the area, at which special meals were provided for the children. The conduct of these area play groups was the responsibility of a group of young volunteer mothers of the particular area, who rotated in their work with the children. They had very short periods of training by the community health workers, supported by others of the health team. This enabled them to initiate these centers, and regular visits by health team members ensured an increasingly higher level of functioning in these play groups.

One of the main purposes of the play groups was to organize health care for the children, including regular health examinations, immunizations, treatments of common infections and injuries, and special feeding. All this was done with special reference to the health education of the children and their mothers, such as provision of simple, inexpensive nutritious foods, growing of vegetables, and personal hygiene of children to prevent common skin and eye infections.

Schoolchildren. The school health service, which was one of the first activities of the health center included:

Periodic health examinations of the children, with emphasis on growth in height and weight, maturation and nutritional status, skin, eye and ear infections, personal cleanliness, detection of the less common abnormalities, and disability.

Dietary surveys were carried out by 24-hour recall of foods eaten. This was done daily with each child for over a period of 1 week, and in one school during four seasons of the year.

Health education was conducted for both teachers and for children. Sessions of direct relevance to the health of the children were organized for various classes at the schools. These included talks by community health workers, discussions and practical demonstrations using field microscopes and other equipment, as well as illustrations and observation visits in the area. A special teaching discussion group, of teachers from various schools and health center staff, was held periodically at the health center.

Action included planting vegetable gardens at each school, which provided part of a school meal prepared by the children. Pit latrines and pits for making compost from waste were constructed at several of the schools, and where possible, water sources were protected from contamination.

These activities were reinforced by a special weekly nutrition clinic held at the health center, with group discussions, demonstrations, and participation in vegetable gardening, poultry keeping, and methods of preparing and cooking various dishes. These sessions were for schoolchildren and those not attending school. It soon became apparent that while nutrition was a subject of importance for the children, special efforts were needed to make it interesting to them. We, therefore, introduced a number of play activities, which rapidly grew into a weekly "Children's Day" at the health center, for which we constructed a sports field for football and other games. The large numbers of children involved became important health educators of their own families, reinforcing the home visits of the community health workers. The discussions between children and their parents resulted in several novel approaches to modernization of common traditional beliefs about the nature of disease. The entire health team was involved in the different facets of these children's activities, with participation of teachers of the various area schools.

Periodic Health Examinations
and Family Health Reviews

An approach to preventive health care of adults was initiated by the introduction of periodic health examinations. Many were referred after treatment at the general curative clinic and others, especially women, came after having been through pre- and postnatal care at the center. These sessions included anthropometry, clinical examinations, laboratory tests, and discussions on traditional and modern concepts of health, and the person's perceptions of his or her own health or that of other family members.

When several members of the family had been examined in one or other of the services, and after their homes had been visited by community health workers, the data were brought together in the form of a family diagnosis and discussed by the health team. The family was invited to a conference on the health of the various members, the care program advised for different individuals and how it was to be carried out, together with consideration of family activities that might contribute to the family's health.

Field Activities

Field work was mainly confined to development of community health programs in the defined area. The expansion of the defined area by extension to homes in adjacent areas demanded different kinds of activities. The initial information needed about the newly added homes was different from the well-established system of health surveillance in neighborhoods that had been incorporated within the defined area for 5 or 10 years. Not only was the data-gathering process different, but the programs of health education and community organization differed in content and in level of sophistication of the families. Community participation was more developed in the older areas, as evidenced by a number of activities, from participation in community health surveillance through supervision of children in preschool child play centers, cooperative endeavor in protection of water sources from pollution, home gardening, and establishing a local market. Each year the new group of homes included in the defined area was introduced to the possibilities offered by the new approach to community health care, not only in terms of the clinic service they were using, but also in terms of their own role in building the program.

The mapping of homesteads in the expanding area and the gathering of demographic information eventually provided us with detailed knowledge of wider kinship networks, which contributed to our understanding of the social and cultural setting of much illness in the community. There were also occasions when we needed a broader type of family interview, in which members of the larger kin lineage group were involved. This ranged from material help to members of one's kin to discussing the epidemiology of tuberculosis and understanding the impact of kin relationships and tensions on the health state of different members.

Thus, apart from the control of outbreaks of epidemic diseases over a very wide region, the field work of the team was focused on the defined area, in which there was intensive health surveillance, health education, and community development. This involved visits to homes and schools in the area and many meetings with formal and informal groups of the community.

Surveys of Health-Related Behavior and the Environment.   As indicated earlier, the community health surveys included an ongoing system of building up knowledge about health-related behavior and the environment. These included KAP (knowledge, attitudes, and practices) studies of:

Seasonal and food production by different homesteads, food storage, gathering and use of wild greens, dietary habits, and methods of cooking.

Infant rearing and feeding practices.

Disposal of refuse and human excreta.

Gathering and storage of water, mapping water supply sources and tests of their purity.

Information on medical care in the community in case of illness, with special emphasis on use of traditional practitioners and the methods used by these practitioners in diagnosis and treatment.

Family and Community Health Education.   While all of us were acutely aware of our role as health educators, and the people were encouraged to discuss health or any other subject they wished, the main function of the community health workers was seen as that of health education and community organization. In addition to general health education, specific programs of education were decided upon from time to time. Programs of education concerned with nutrition and communicable diseases were directed toward the needs of individual families and the community as a whole. Examples of the main topics were:

Nutrition

The relationship between food and health, especially for the pregnant and nursing mother.

Growth and development through infancy and childhood.

Kwashiorkor, marasmus, and pellagra. Appreciation of the causes, home treatment, and prevention.

The control of communicable diseases

Syphilis, with special reference to the role of the migrant worker in the epidemiology of syphilis. Hence the need for effective treatment.

Tuberculosis. Emphasis on the traditional interpretation of this disease, which was not related to the concept of transmission.

Gastroenteritis in young children, and the enteric diseases.

Sanitary disposal of refuse, protection of water supplies and food.

Education and assistance in the protection of water sources, making compost pits or heaps, and constructing pit latrines.

Fly control was very difficult, but protection of food from flies was practicable.

Boiling drinking-water.

Personal cleanliness in protection against common skin diseases from infection, such as scabies and impetigo contagiosa. This was associated with demonstrations of ways of treating the whole family.

Community Development

Our approach was promotion of health in a broad sense, including activities directed toward increasing the attendance of children at school, improving agricultural and home gardening methods, and establishing play centers for preschool children of different neighborhoods. There they would have special enriched meals with various locally produced vegetables, including the soya bean, introduced by the health center, and milk supplements.

Community participation and involvement in decision making was encouraged, since without it many of the activities could not have taken place. Thus, as mentioned, the supervisors of the play centers were voluntary workers. The home gardening and agricultural program was carried further by the formation of a club, concerned in the first instance with cooperative buying of seeds and extending to the purchase of implements. As these programs developed, an increasing number of homes were able to sell produce. A market was established to which men and women brought their produce for sale, and at the request of the market committee it was agreed that it could be held at the health center. Arising from this, a women's club was formed, the initial activities of which were baking, cooking, sewing, knitting, and gardening. Members of the club were encouraged by one of the tribal chiefs to represent women of the area at his meetings, and to advise the health center.

Another community activity was the protection of water supplies. Surveys carried out by the community health workers indicated that groups of homes had common sources for collecting water. These were usually springs, which we had tested for purity at the source. Protection of these water supplies was undertaken by groups of men from the homes concerned.

EVALUATION OF
THE VARIOUS PROGRAMS

This was one of the functions of the health team, involving weekly reviews of activities and continuing surveillance of the community's health. Some of the more important activities involved the setting up of our own health information system, on the basis of which we evaluated different aspects of the combined community medicine and primary health care.

The Health Information System
of the Health Center

The intensive activities which we developed with the families and the community in the defined area itself, and with people from this area who came to the health center, led us to formulate our approach on the following lines:

To coordinate care of individuals in the clinics of the health center with intervention directed toward changing health-related behavior of families and the community.

To carry out social, behavioral, and epidemiologic investigations for community diagnosis, as the foundation for intervention programs.

To organize an ongoing system of surveillance of the extent to which we were doing what we had decided to do, and evaluation of the various programs, by measurement of changes in community behavior and of the state of health of the community.

This required the development of a system of recording which would readily provide information on the health of the community, factors known to determine its state of health, and relevant data on the health center's activities.

Community diagnosis and the surveillance of health and health-related behavior required:

1. Demographic information. We established a system of gathering data on all families in the defined area, starting with an area of 130 homes and extending to 1300 homes with a population of 10,500, over a 15-year period (1942 to 1957). At the same time we introduced an unofficial system of birth and death registration at the health center, in cooperation with the various neighborhood communities and their leaders. In- and out-migration of individuals was reported and recorded, as was the settling in of a new family or the departure of another. We thus had available basic denominator and numerator data of the following kinds:
   Population, according to age, sex, education, occupation, marital status, kinship networks
   Pregnancies, live- and stillbirths
   Deaths
   Migration into and out of the area
2. Determinants of health. There was little or no relevant information available on this area, and we therefore carried out such special surveys as the following:

The social structure, especially kinship and family responsibility for health promotion, care of the sick, and other health-relevant actions.

Work and social activities of men and women, including the construction of a calendar of seasonal variation in these activities.

Nutrition. Seasonal dietary surveys of special groups, such as infant feeding practices, diet of school children, dietary customs in pregnancy. Food production surveys: annual measurement of main crops, seasonal studies of home vegetable gardens and milk production, sample studies of ownership of livestock and poultry, food storage and cooking methods.

Housing and the environment. Detailed survey of each homestead including various structures and their use; water supply points, mapping of springs used by families of various neighborhoods during different seasons, with study of their purity and potential for protection; disposal of animal and human refuse and excreta.

Traditional concepts about health and disease, in relation to use of services.

Utilization of the health center's services.

3. Health and morbidity. The greatest amount of material gathered in this respect was from the team's clinical and survey records. Clinic records were filed in family folders, and all acute diseases were noted on special forms, which were kept by the doctors in their consulting rooms. Extraction of these data was made by the doctors themselves, allowing for epidemiologic surveillance of infectious diseases and syndromes of acute nutritional failure. Clinical and field records were periodically summarized for each family and abstracted for analysis of health indices, such as mortality and morbidity rates, immunization rates, physical growth, and nutritional status. These were related to various measurements of health-related behavior and environment of the families and community as a whole. The information service maintained by the health center team enabled us to analyze change over the years.

The Weekly Team Conference

Perhaps the most important institution we established for exchange of health information between members of the team was the weekly staff conference, attended by all the community health workers, nurses, medical aides, and doctors. Later, when we trained our own health recorders, they became central figures in these conferences. These were very busy and rewarding sessions, with active participation by all in the interchange of information about activities at the health center itself and in the community. The various activities were summarized and recorded at these meetings. In respect to the population in the defined area, the records allowed for abstraction about each family and the community's health. The summary included:

Attendances at the Health Center
For general curative purposes, as well as pre- and postnatal supervision and treatment; well-baby sessions focusing on growth and development; treatment of syphilis, which had a very high prevalence at the time.

Home Visiting by Community Health Workers in the Defined Area
Follow-up visits for advice and discussion about personal health care
Health surveillance: routine data collection and special surveys
Health education and action

Other Activities
School visits, meetings with various groups
Investigation and control of reported epidemics
Significant events

In the early years, a diary was kept of the proceedings and reports of these meetings. This proved of immense value in administration and decision making. A summary of some entries at one of the weekly conferences is presented.

Attendances at the Health Center

	Total Attendances for the Week	Prenatal	Well-Baby Session	Syphilis Treatment
All patients	665	45	24	279
Patients living in defined area	255	14	24	97
Percent of total attendance	38	31	100	35

Home Visiting by Community Health Workers to Homes in the Defined Area

Total homes visited	212
Purpose of visits (a single visit often had several purposes)	
Follow-up visits in regard to personal health care at the health center	118
Health surveillance—routine and special surveys	64
Health education and action	111

Reports for Analysis of Vital Statistics and Demography

Births	5
deaths	11
marriage	1
pregnancy	4
census of homes	7
population changes in 6 homes, migration of workers: to the city from home	4
return home from city	5

An illustration of one community health program, and its evaluation, is presented in Chapter 9.

REFERENCES

1. Djukanovic V, Mach EP (eds): Alternative Approaches to Meeting Basic Health Needs in Developing Countries. Geneva, WHO, 1975
2. Newell KW (ed): Health by the People. Geneva, WHO, 1975
3. World Health Organization: Report on International Conference on Primary Health Care. Alma-Ata. Geneva—New York, WHO, 1978
4. Bennett FJ: Primary health care and developing countries. Soc Sci Med 13A:505, 1979
5. ——: Mortality in a rural Zulu community. Br J Prev Soc Med 14:1, 1960
6. Gluckman H (chairman): Report of the National Health Services Commission. Pretoria, Government Printer, 1944
7. Kark SL: A health service among the rural Bantu. S Afr Med J 16:197, 1942
8. ——: A health unit as family doctor and health adviser. S Afr Med J 18:39,1944
9. ——, Kark E: A practice of social medicine. Clin Proc 4:284, 1945
10. Gale GW: Health centre practice. S Afr Med J 20:326, 1946
11. Kark SL: Health centre service. In Cluver EH (ed): Social Medicine. Central News Agency S.A., 1951, Chap 26
12. ——, Cassel J: The Polela Health Centre. S Afr Med J 26:101, 131, 1952
13. ——: Nutrition and Adjustment in the Changing Society of Polela. Doctoral thesis. Univ. Witwatersrand Library, 1953
14. Cassel J: A comprehensive health program among South African Zulus. In Paul BD (ed): Health, Culture and Community. New York, Russell Sage Foundation, 1955, p 15
15. Kark SL, Steuart GW (eds): A Practice of Social Medicine. Edinburgh, Livingstone, 1962
16. Slome C: Community health in rural Polela. In Kark SL, Steuart GW (eds): A Practice of Social Medicine. Edinburgh, Livingstone, 1962, p 280
17. Kark SL: Community Health Care in Developing Countries. In Frederiksen HS: Epidemographic Surveillance. Chapel Hill, Carolina Population Center. Monograph 13, 1971

CHAPTER 9

COMMUNITY-ORIENTED PRIMARY HEALTH CARE OF INFANTS IN RURAL POLELA

Of the many functions that women fulfill in Polela, none were regarded as more important than that of childbearing and subsequent rearing. Both men and women expressed a strong desire for children, and it was seldom that anyone wished to limit the size of the family. Complaints of sterility were very common, even in women who had borne as many as four children but had not been pregnant for several years. Spacing of births was related to several factors: the traditional abstention from sexual intercourse during the period of breast feeding, which was still observed to a limited extent; the absence of men from their homes for prolonged periods while at work in the cities; and in a few cases, contraception. Advice on family spacing was rarely sought, and then only by the few more educated women.

A woman usually had her first baby at her maiden home, with her own mother being the birth attendant, or possibly some older woman of the neighborhood known for her experience. Subsequent babies were commonly born in her married home. Until the advent of the health center, there were no qualified midwives practicing in the area.

Following a successful birth, the mother began her long process of infant nurture. The average Polela mother breast-fed her baby for some 18 to 24 months. Thus, the whole process of childbirth, from conception until complete weaning from the breast, extended over a period of 2 to 3 years. This fact, together with the high fertility rate, explained an outstanding feature of the role of women in Polela society. At any one time, some 30 percent of women of childbearing age,

Dr. Emily Kark is co-author of this chapter.

15 to 45 years, and over 50 percent of those aged 20 to 35 years were involved in a direct physiologic and intimate association with an infant, expected or born. Mothers, young and middle-aged, were to be seen at work or other activities with their babies tied on their backs.

THE INITIAL CASE FOR ACTION

The case for initiating a special community-wide program for the promotion of infant health, with preventive and curative components, was manifest very soon after the center was initiated. Our impressions of health status and morbidity in early childhood were formed during the first 2 years of experience at the general clinic, which was opened very soon after the establishment of the health center. This walk-in clinic became well known to people near and far, mothers and their young children making up a large proportion of the patients. The commonest diagnoses in children during their first 2 years of life were severe cases of gastroenteritis, upper respiratory infections, acute bronchitis, pneumonia, failure to grow, and marked malnutrition. Many infants had generalized scabies with superimposed impetigo.

We were impressed by the large numbers of cases who were under the care of traditional practitioners. The management of diarrhea in infants illustrates the extent to which traditional concepts about disease determined the family's actions. The community's perception of diarrhea in infants varied according to the accompanying physical signs. Severe diarrhea, with green stools and undigested curds, was a signal for the diagnosis of a particular, severe condition known locally as *isolo*. A sunken anterior fontanelle was regarded as a specific diagnostic sign; skin rashes, varying from mild impetiginous lesions to extensive infected dermatoses, added severity to the prognosis for the child's survival.

The importance of a diagnosis of *isolo* was not its similarity to gastroenteritis associated with dehydration and other signs of nutritional failure, but rather the community's concept of its etiology. It was considered by the people to be a disease transmitted by the mother, both congenitally and through breast feeding. Mothers were believed to have been affected by an ill-wisher, who had directed her by supernatural means to a place struck by lightning. The traditional practitioner's actions were aimed at treatment of the diarrhea and prevention of the cause. The former involved such treatments as enemas using grass reeds, and the latter advice to stop breast feeding. both interventions often aggravated the condition, and it was at this stage that the baby was usually brought to the health center.

Once the mother believed that her breast milk was a cause of the baby's illness, she could not be expected to listen to advice that she should continue breast feeding. And yet this was very important for a baby's survival, since there were no adequate substitutes for breast milk in this community. This was an obvious case for health education and for the establishment of an understanding relationship between the health team and mothers.

Notwithstanding this belief system, community leaders and older women were eager for the health center to focus on the problem, and in so doing be especially concerned with the health of children and their mothers. We therefore decided to make this aspect a major feature of the health center's activities. The program that was developed will be reviewed here along the following lines:

1. Community diagnosis and health surveillance, by which we sought to answer questions on the state of health of infants in the community and the factors determining their health.
2. Action. What was being done by the community itself, and by various health and other agencies? Could anything be done to improve the situation? In answering, we will focus on the activities of the health center team and the community.
3. Evaluation of the program, including its effects on infant health in this community.

Each of these aspects was an ongoing process, community diagnosis and health surveillance proceeding along with action and evaluation measures. As far as possible, the decisions made on educational and clinical programs were based on the knowledge being gained by the accumulation and analysis of data on health and its determinants.

COMMUNITY DIAGNOSIS AND HEALTH SURVEILLANCE

In order to answer questions as to the state of infant health and its determinants, we required basic information on the population, which was not available in Polela. There was no accurate census, nor was there any record of births and deaths. We were able to achieve this in the framework of our decision to establish a more intensive program of family and community health care. This involved the health team in establishing a defined area of homes for health surveillance, health education, and practical assistance to families and other community groups, in action programs of health relevance. Following the first year of this approach, additional groups of homes were included in the health center's defined area. Each was a natural geographic area of homes along a mountain slope. As each area of homes was included, a system of gathering demographic information was instituted. This involved:

Initial Household Census.   This was done by community health workers conducting systematic surveys of all homes in the area. It included the name, sex, estimated date of birth, education, occupation, and relationship to head of household of each household member. This was updated through reports of births, deaths, and in- and out-movements.

Birth Recording.   This was based on information obtained from the health center's prenatal records, notifications by the community health workers, and by the families. The record included details about the mother and baby:

> Mother: Name, age, address, marital status, parity, prenatal care, place of delivery, birth attendant, and comment on labor.
> Baby: Name, sex, birth date, rank, live or stillbirth, condition at birth, birthplace.

Death Reporting.   This was based on information from several sources, the clinic records, community health workers, and the community itself. The death record we maintained included: name of the deceased, age, sex, address, cause of death, date and place of death.

Gathering this demographic information enabled us to calculate various health indices. Those of direct relevance to infancy were: birth rates, live- and stillbirth rates per 1000 population, infant mortality rates, neonatal and postneonatal mortality rates per 100 live births.

In addition, the household census provided data for the infant population in respect of total number and distribution according to sex, birth rank, and spacing from the previous child.

The annual expansion of the defined area provided the opportunity to compare a number of health indices, including infant mortality rates in the different areas, according to the length of time each had been incorporated into the defined area. Thus, each new area became a control population for the areas previously included. This provided a very useful way of evaluating community health programs. An example is presented later in this chapter.

Data Gathering

We had to build a system of gathering data on infant health and its determinants in this community, since there was almost no measurable information available from other sources. The main activities at the health center, namely, treatment of sick infants and the well-baby session, allowed us to build up a body of information on infant health, analyzable in morbidity rates, as well as growth and development, with special emphasis on weight gain through the first year. Similarly, the clinical activities at the health center, when recorded in relation to the defined area population, provided some of the information needed concerning determinants of infant health, such as health of mothers through pregnancy and lactation and infant feeding practices.

In addition to the information obtained at the clinics of the health center, much attention was given to the collection of data in the field. This was the responsibility of the community health workers, who were specially trained by us for such epidemographic surveillance and studies of health-relevant behavior. This kind of intensive health surveillance, through ongoing household surveys, can be carried out only with the acceptance of such workers by the community, which, in turn, is part of the relationship between community and health center.

The data gathered by the field workers were complemented by that of the clinics and other activities at the health center itself.

Community diagnosis of infant health and disease, and the determining factors, are considered here in respect of:

1. Birth and death rates, morbidity rates of selected diseases, and weight growth.
2. Measurements of reproductive and family formation factors influencing infant health:
   fertility rates, mother's age at birth of baby, birth rank, maternal health through pregnancy: nutrition, syphilis, and care through pregnancy and confinement.
3. Measurements of health-relevant behavior: infant feeding practices, utilization of health center services.

Some Measurements of Infant Health

Infant Mortality. Our first impression of a very high mortality rate in infancy was confirmed by the early mortality rates calculated for babies born in the defined area. In our first defined area of 132 homes, with 887 persons, 40 babies were born during the year, and there were 11 deaths in infants under 1 year. In the succeeding early years of the program, each additional area incorporated into the health center's defined area had similar high infant mortality rates. With 199 live births recorded in the first year of inclusion of new areas over the initial 3 years, the IMR was 26 percent. This will be reviewed in more detail in the evaluation of the program.

The accumulation of birth and death records allowed for the analysis of stillbirth, neonatal (0 to 4 weeks), and postneonatal (4 weeks to 1 year) mortality rates, as well as the total IMR (Table 9-1). The stillbirth rate, and both the neonatal and postneonatal mortality rates, were very high.

The case for an intensive program to reduce infant mortality was clear. Further investigation of the causes of death was carried out while we were implementing a care program.

Morbidity. Following through a group of children over a period of 5 years provided information on morbidity in infancy and early childhood. There were 146 children born in this period in one of the geographic districts of the defined area; the average duration of the follow-up was over 3 years. Although the health center had these children under fairly frequent observation, the clinical records were not a full reflection of their total disease experience. The incidence of diagnosed common diseases in these children is shown in Table 9-2.

Gastroenteritis, scabies with impetigo, and severe upper respiratory infections were very common, and recurrences were frequent. Upper respiratory infections were frequently complicated by pneumonia and otitis media. The rapidity with which this occurrred was sufficient to warrant careful supervision of these children. Added to this was the likelihood of an associated diarrhea, which commonly precipitated acute nutritional failure. Diseases such as whooping cough, measles, and epidemic acute conjunctivitis were common and

TABLE 9-1

The Accumulated Stillbirth and Infant Mortality Rate over the First
Four-Year Period of the Health Center's Defined Area

	LIVE BIRTHS	STILLBIRTHS*	NEONATAL DEATHS†	POST-NEONATAL DEATHS†	IMR†
Number	794	35	48	105	153
Rate, percent		4.2	6.0	13.2	19.3

*Stillbirth rate: Number of stillbirths per 100 total births (stillbirths and live births).
†These rates are expressed as the number of deaths in the total 4-year period per 100 live births in the same period.

TABLE 9-2

The Incidence of Common Diseases Diagnosed in a Group of 146 Infants and Children Followed over a Five-Year Period

| | CHILDREN | |
	Number	Percentage
Acute gastroenteritis	70	48
Skin infections	60	41
Upper respiratory infections	62	42
Acute otitis media	17	12
Pneumonia	22	15
Whooping cough	27	18
Measles	14	10
Acute conjunctivitis (epidemic)	30	21
Accidents and injuries	24	16
Children born to mothers diag- nosed to have syphilis	30	21
Children in whom no illness was diagnosed during the period	10	7

serious maladies, precipitating severe malnutrition as well as the more usually recognized complications of pneumonia, otitis media, and eye diseases. The high proportion of babies, 20 percent, born of mothers having a positive serologic test for syphilis during pregnancy presented a major problem. They seldom manifested the classical signs of congenital syphilis, but presented a difficult problem, as they failed to grow satisfactorily and had a higher incidence of the acute illnesses mentioned.

The nutritional effects of these conditions were among the most important complications. The common occurrence of gastroenteritis especially had an adverse influence on nutritional status and growth. Acute nutritional failure, kwashiorkor or marasmus, was frequently precipitated by these acute illnesses. Malnutrition, as expressed by a relative failure to grow, is the background on which this happened, the acute illness changing the low-grade or chronic condition of malnutrition to an acute nutritional failure syndrome, like florid kwashiorkor or marasmus.

In Polela children, the acute mucous membrane reaction, which is a feature of measles, would frequently be followed by an exaggeration of such common signs of malnutrition as glossitis, gingivitis, and cheilosis, and the acute conjunctivitis associated with an episode of measles was commonly followed by chronic conjunctivitis and blepharitis. These last lesions were also noted during a "pink eye" (acute conjunctivitis) epidemic among the children. Whooping cough was even more dramatic in its impact on their clinical nutritional status. This important relationship between infection and malnutrition has been recognized for many years. In the early years of this century, McCarrison stated that infection may not only "precipitate the onset of symptoms due to food deficiency" but it might "import new clinical features to the food deficiency syndrome."[1]

Growth in Weight of Moderately Well Babies. The routine weighing of babies at the general curative clinic indicated that a considerable number were markedly underweight for their age. With the objective of preparing a growth chart for use by the nurses as a standard for the babies of this community, it was decided to analyze the weight growth of moderately well babies. Reference has been made to the well-baby session conducted at the health center. Among the infants referred to this clinic were a number who could be classified as moderately well, using the following criteria:

Mother's Health. To the best of our knowledge, she had had a normal pregnancy and labor, with no evidence of syphilis (serologic test), tuberculosis, severe malnutrition, or other disorders. There were very few expectant mothers without some clinical signs of malnutrition. Babies of mothers whose nutritional state was not markedly below the average were included in this analysis.

Family Health. A history of one or more recent cases of tuberculosis in the home, including primary infections in infants, excluded a baby from this analysis.

Baby's Health. Any infant with signs of congenital disorder, including congenital syphilis, was excluded, as were all babies who had any severe illness during their first year of life. This excluded those who had whooping cough, pneumonia, acute otitis media, severe diarrhea, primary tuberculous infection, and acute nutritional failure.

For Polela the criteria were highly selective, with only 98 babies being selected of the several thousand seen during the first 4 years of the practice. The findings were compared with black and white American middle-class babies of that period.[2]

During the first 3 months, the Polela babies were found to compare favorably with the United States babies, the mean weight at 3 months being 12.56 lb (5.71 kg). By the age of 6 months, while still growing fairly well, the mean weight being 15.77 lb (7.17 kg), the Polela babies were lighter than those of the United States at this age. By 9 months, mean weight 17.65 lb (8.02 kg), and even more so at 12 months, 18.38 lb (8.35 kg), the Polela babies were markedly retarded when compared with the American babies, who averaged approximately 22 lb at 1 year.

The Polela findings constituted a baseline for evaluation of progress in subsequent years. This will be discussed in more detail later in this chapter.

Some Measurements of Reproduction and Family Formation

Defining the main factors responsible for the poor state of health, as reflected in the high infant mortality rate and the high incidence and prevalence of illness and malnutrition in infancy, is an epidemiologic exercise of considerable complexity. In a community such as Polela, birth rank, family size, parity of the mother, maternal age, and birth spacing are associated with other features of the society, namely, poverty, lack of food, social disorganization, lack of education, poor sanitation, and lack of modern public health and medical services. The interdependence of these various factors was not analyzed in the community diagnosis of infant health in Polela. Instead, we have analyzed the prevalence of the various factors that are considered to be determinants of health, as found in a variety of worldwide studies. For a review of these, and for studies focusing on developing countries, the World Health Organization collaborative study on family formation and health is helpful.[3]

Birth Rate, Age of Mother, and Birth Rank.   Large families, and the familiar sight of pregnant women and mothers carrying babies on their backs, were indications of a high fertility rate in this community. The birth reporting introduced by the health center confirmed this impression. The average live birth rate was 40.6 per 1000 population during the first 4 years, and remained at that level 8 years later.

The fertility rates were high in all age groups, one in every five women, aged 20 to 35 years, having a baby per year. Births to teenage mothers constituted no less than 17 percent of the total births, and those to mothers over 35 years of age, a further 13 percent. While a large proportion of births were first-born, 31 percent, there were a considerable number of high-birth-rank babies, 38 percent rank 4 and over (Table 9–3).

Marital Status of Mothers.   Traditional Zulu mores frowned very severely on unmarried motherhood, but the social disorganization of societies such as Polela led to a reluctant acceptance of the reality.

TABLE 9-3
Selected Reproductive Indices of Relevance to Infant Health

Fertility Rates

Age of women (years)	10–14	15–19	20–24	25–29	30–34	35–39	40–49
Number	453	417	394	316	266	214	369
% with live birth in a year	0.7	11	19	23	19	13	2

Distribution of 284 Births According to Age of Mother

Age of mother (years)	<20	20–24	25–29	30–34	35–39	40+
%	17.3	26.5	26.2	17.7	9.5	2.8

Birth Rank of the Babies

Rank	1	2	3	4	5	6+
% of babies	30.6	14.3	16.7	12.8	9.7	15.9

Girls engaged to be married, having babies fathered by the man whom they subsequently married, were socially acceptable. The tradition of the levirate continued, and widowed women bearing children by their late husband's brother were thus acceptable. Of the births recorded, no less than 11.5 percent were born to unmarried mothers (excluding those mothers just referred to). As would be expected, the highest proportion of these were first births. In fact, 30 percent of all reported first births and over 10 percent of second- and third-rank births were children of unmarried mothers.

Maternal Health in Pregnancy. A considerable proportion of babies were born with a heritage of maternal malnutrition and venereal disease, especially syphilis.

Maternal malnutrition was manifest in a number of nonspecific clinical signs of the skin and mucous membranes. Follicular hyperkeratosis (phrynoderma), dry and cracked skin, occasional pellagra dermatosis, angular stomatitis, cheilosis, and glossitis were common, as were blepharitis and conjunctival changes. Of interest was the almost complete absence of anemia in pregnancy. The most striking feature of malnutrition in expectant mothers was the relative failure in weight gain through pregnancy. An analysis was carried out of the weight changes of a selected group of relatively normal or well women attending the prenatal clinics of the health center. Outstanding findings of this analysis were:[4,5]

The average total increase in weight through pregnancy was 9.5 lb (4.32 kg)

During the first 4 weeks 35 percent gained over 1 lb (above 650 gm) and 42 percent lost over 1 lb

During the last month: 52 percent gained more than 1 lb

The analysis involved a limited number of women, 116 in all, and the findings must, therefore, be interpreted with caution. However, the limited change in weight during pregnancy was consistent with studies of height and weight of men and women in the community carried out over the same period of time.[4] Positive features were the almost complete absence of diabetes mellitus and ischemic heart disease and the rarity of hypertensive disease in pregnancy.

Syphilis in Pregnancy. The rate of syphilis, mainly latent syphilis, in the pregnant women using the health center was 35 percent, as assessed by the serologic tests used at the time. This, no doubt, represented an accumulation of untreated disease over many years of social pathology.[6] The outcome of pregnancy in mothers diagnosed to have syphilis was found to be poorer than expected. Stillbirths were reported in 8.9 percent of 270 such mothers, as compared with 3.4 percent in 1357 mothers with negative serologic tests for syphilis.

The Family and Infant Health

Over and above the reproductive factors and the mother's state of health, illness in other members of the family was important. This was especially so for the many infectious diseases transmitted to babies by other children in the home, fathers, grandparents, and other kin. A common problem was presented by the return home from the city of a sick migrant worker. We had early warning of this when, shortly after the establishment of the health center, a young married man returned home from his work in the city. He was very ill and had come back so that he might die at home. The family decided that he was suffering from *isifuba sedliso* ("poisoning" of the chest, thought to be introduced through food or beer by an ill-wisher), and that he should be treated by a traditional practitioner. The health center was not consulted, but a community health worker visiting this home in the course of his routine work saw the patient and noted his severe illness. He suspected pulmonary tuberculosis, discussed the desirability of care by the health center, and brought a specimen of sputum for laboratory examination. Tubercle bacilli were found, and yet another home was added to the growing number known to have had an active case of tuberculosis.

In the third week after his return home, the man died. The importance of the single positive sputum finding emerged within a relatively short time. His death was followed by the deaths of four infants and young children of this homestead, within 2 years. Positive tuberculin tests confirmed primary tuberculous infection, associated with advanced malnutrition, with kwashiorkor diagnosed in two of the four children.

Other family factors that were no doubt of considerable importance in determining the health of infants were: extreme poverty, sometimes with hunger and starvation, ignorance and superstition, insanitary home conditions, inadequate personal hygiene, and social disorganization in family living. The last was a product of migration of men to the towns for work. This was not merely a result of the attraction of the city for this peasant population, but a necessity in the face of poverty at home.

Migrant Labor. For several generations, Polela men had been involved in a process of migration to the towns for work, and it was expected that a young man would look to a future of extended periods of work in a city, while his family remained at home. The average man spent a considerable part of his adult life away from home, starting in his late teens and continuing after marriage into middle age and beyond, when his children were passing through their infancy, childhood, and adolescence. Men were away for periods of 9 to 15 months, and sometimes longer. They might come home several times a year for short visits, usually for ploughing their fields, but more often they remained away for long periods of time. A survey of this was undertaken by the health center, with startling results. The percentage of men away at work for at least 1 month during the year of the study varied according to age:

15–19 years	47%
20–34 years	84%
35–49 years	62%
50 and over	32%

Thus, many babies were born and reared in homes without men, except for the occasional visits home by the working men, and those limited numbers who worked in the area or were too old or disabled to go away. The burden of home management and food production, infant care and childrearing, fell on the mothers and grandmothers, with the help of their younger sons and daughters. Decision making at times of illness or other crises was difficult, and often postponed until contact was made with the menfolk in town. This could mean medical neglect in cases of need, and was especially critical in infancy.

Measurements of Health-Related Behavior

Breast Feeding. Investigation of home care of the newborn indicated that breast feeding was not initiated until a free flow of milk had replaced colostrum, usually between the third to the fifth day after birth. We conducted this investigation because of our early observation of an apparently high incidence of diarrhea in early infancy. As all the babies were born at home, this was obviously not the type of neonatal diarrhea known to occur in newborns of nursery units of hospital obstetrics departments.

During the early days after birth, the baby was fed by bottle on boiled water and a cereal drink, usually made with maize or sorghum.

Although the water was boiled, it was poured into a bottle that was not sterilized. A second common practice was the enema, using a reed. After birth, babies were given an enema to remove the meconium, and this cleaning procedure was continued once or twice daily during the first week; later it remained a feature of treatment for various illnesses in infancy and early childhood.

On enquiry, mothers and grandmothers indicated that the early cereal drink was a relatively recent custom, having been introduced when there was a dearth of cows in milk. We found that it was a soft point in the culture, that is, one that could readily be changed, whereas the enema habit was a hard point and would not be readily forsaken. With this knowledge, we discussed both habits with mothers, focusing on the feeding practice and encouraging earlier initiation of breast feeding. This helped considerably, and the incidence of neonatal diarrhea declined in babies of mothers who had attended the health center for prenatal care. Similar health education of the grandmothers was carried out at home visits. Early on, it became clear that real advance in mothering was best achieved by involving the grandmothers, who directed the care given to babies, especially the firstborns of younger mothers.

While babies were being subjected to the care outlined, their mothers were also having traditional treatment at home. Their breasts were massaged and warm cloths applied to make the milking-off process easier. This treatment was apparently successful in preventing overdistension and tension of breasts, and it was rare for mothers to experience any difficulty in initiating and maintaining satisfactory breast feeding. A health center survey of the prevalence of breast feeding confirmed this impression: At 1 month, 99.4 percent were breast fed, and at 3, 6, 9, and 12 months, the percentage was, respectively, 99, 97, 96, and 84.

We believed that the successful initiation of breast feeding was related not only to the postnatal treatment described, but also to a common practice among young girls, who were encouraged by family and peers to manipulate their breasts and draw out the nipples, from the time of early development of breasts at puberty. This was probably an important factor in hardening the nipples and thus preventing retraction as well as cracked tender nipples in the nursing mother.

Maintenance of Breast Feeding and Weaning to Other Foods. During the early days after birth, mother and baby were confined together in a hut at home, and a very close physical relationship was maintained. Once breast feeding was initiated, the feeding relationship was one of indulgence, mother responding to baby's demands and de-

veloping a sense and feel of when to feed baby. We have used the term
"adjusted feeding relationship" to describe the mother-baby breast
feeding method of Polela, which implies a mutual relationship between
the two. The term "self-demand feeding" refers only to the baby's initiative, thus excluding the important initiating role of the mother. The
process as observed was of a mother who often anticipates her baby's
need for the breast, even before baby demands it by crying.

Breast feeding continued for 15 or more months in the majority of
cases, but not uncommonly it was terminated earlier. We noted that
16 percent of mothers had stopped breast feeding by 12 months.
Among the important causes of this were illness in the baby and
another pregnancy.

The process of weaning to other foods was of much interest, since
the foods to which the babies were weaned were a major determinant
of their failure to grow and of the clinical syndromes of kwashiorkor,
marasmus, and other less severe signs of malnutrition. Together with
infection, they were also responsible for repeated attacks of gastroenteritis. The commonest weaning food was maize, in the form of a
gruel and later in the various maize dishes as prepared for adults.
Milk, or its products, was a preferred weaning food, but was often not
available. Our surveys of milk availability to various homes provided
clear evidence of this fact: Thirty-four percent of the homes in one of
the defined areas possessed no cow, and a further 28 percent had only
one cow. A more realistic picture was presented in a series of studies
we undertook at different seasons over several years. Even in the summer, the best season of the year, only 47 percent of homes had at least
some milk available, and through the winter and early spring only 10
to 20 percent had some milk. Of more than 700 homes surveyed, the
percentage that had no cows in milk at various seasons over a 3-year
period was as follows:

Midsummer	53
Late summer	58
Midwinter	80
Early spring	89

The amount of milk produced by cows in milk was pitifully small,
ranging from the highest average yield of 2 liters per day in the summer to the lowest of one-quarter and one-eighth liters through the
winter and early spring.

Not only was there little milk available, but there was a paucity of
other foods to which infants could be weaned. As previously dis-

cussed, there was widespread severe soil erosion, and consequently the main fields provided poor yields of staple crops, in addition to limited varieties. Within a short time after reaping, there were already insufficient maize, sorghum, and dried beans in the vast majority of homes. The same was true of their home gardens, in which they planted maize and beans with potatoes and pumpkins. A limited number of homes grew additional vegetables, mainly cabbage and sweet potatoes. Poultry was the most common meat available, although it was seldom eaten more than once a week, and eggs were seldom used even in the feeding of infants and young children.

Thus, our early impressions were of infants having only breast milk for 5 or more months, followed by the addition of maize preparations, which seldom included milk. Later the infant ate from the family pot, which might include wild greens and other foods. In addition to this poor diet in the second half of infancy, the baby was exposed to additional hazards of insanitary environs, polluted food and water, and contact with a family of which several members usually had a skin infection or other communicable disease. Open fires and smoke-filled huts, especially in the extremely cold winters of this mountainous countryside, added to the hazards of infancy.

Summary of Community Diagnosis of Infant Health

To summarize the community diagnosis of infant health, the major features were a very high infant mortality rate, resulting mainly from preventable and treatable disease, and malnutrition. The main determinants of this were found to be the following risk factors:

Reproductive factors: high birth and fertility rates, large families, relatively high proportion of teenage and unmarried mothers.

Maternal health: widespread malnutrition, high prevalence of syphilis.

Family health: high prevalence of acute and chronic infectious diseases, associated with:

Extreme poverty, often with lack of food.

Ignorance and superstition.

Poor hygiene of the environs and person.

Social disorganization, with fathers away from home for prolonged periods.

Infant feeding practices:

Negative features, early neonatal feeding with cereal drinks before initiation of breast feeding; weaning foods, predominantly maize.

An outstanding positive feature was the successful initiation and maintenance of breast feeding, associated with continuing close contact between mother and baby.

Health Care. The traditional home remedies used, and utilization of traditional practitioners, often led to harmful delay in seeking more effective treatment, as well as causing iatrogenic complications.

INTERVENTION AND EVALUATION
OF ACTION PROGRAMS

The community was aware of the fact that there was much illness, especially in mothers and children. Their perception of the nature of these illnesses, their customary practices, and the place of the traditional practitioner have been briefly described.

The advent of the health center in this community introduced an agency among the main functions of which was health education. Had its functions been restricted to providing a general curative service meeting the needs of the sick who sought its help, the center might have had a significant effect on individual medical care but a restricted influence on the health of this changing society. Health education and community organization became a foundation for a unified practice of community medicine and primary care, thus developing an integrated promotive, preventive, and curative service.

An important focus of the health center's practice was that of education for healthy living. As a health project that had an educational orientation, it was concerned with what the people in the community felt, thought, and did about health. Thus, in addition to health examinations of individuals and observations of health-relevant behavior at home, discussions with individuals, families, and other groups were a feature of the health center programs. By associating observations and discussions we were able to determine some of the more important felt and unfelt needs of the community and individual families. Being informal, the discussions ranged over a wide field of interests and problems with which people were concerned. These discussions were the foundation of the educational program. A common subject was, as expected, sickness and its nature, with doctors, medical aides, nurses, and community health workers encouraging the individual or group to express attitudes and worries. In this way, the varying concepts of the people were discussed and related to modern knowledge. A relationship of mutual respect between the health center team and the community developed, and it was common for patients or families to discuss their worries, family problems, or the nature of illness, whether thought to be due to natural or supernatural causes.

The change that was taking place in the concepts of the people was a fundamental process in which health education had an important role to play.

The general aims of the intervention program were:

Reduction of infant mortality.

Treatment of sick children.

Prevention of disease.

Promotion of improved growth and nutritional status.

Encouragement of existing infant rearing and feeding practices where promotive of health, and their modification where indicated.

To achieve these general aims, more specific objectives were gradually defined as we learned more about the health problems, the community's behavior, and infant rearing practices, and as our own skills in community health care developed. The specific objectives had to be related to the actual situation, which was extremely unfavorable. In retrospect, this was as unlikely a setting as any could be for the achievement of significant change in the stated aims. This was not only because of the poverty and social disorganization in the community, but also because the health center's program was not part of general social policy.

The specific objectives will be outlined in detail together with the intervention programs and their evaluation. The infant health program was a very important part of community health action. Like the other community medicine programs, it involved activities at the health center itself, in the people's homes, at schools and churches, in the few shops, at water-gathering points, and in the home gardens and cultivated fields of the various families. The nature of the home visits and group discussions, conducted mainly by the community health workers, will first be described, followed by a review of several important aspects of the infant health program.

The Home Visit

The home visit by a community health worker was different from that of doctors, medical aides, or nurses. It was an integral and fundamental part of community health education. The aim was to be accepted in all homes regardless of the presence or absence of illness. The initial visits were at the initiative of the community health worker, and later often at the initiative of the family or a group for meeting at a particular home. The frequency with which the health worker would visit various homes in a neighborhood was influenced by the wishes of the families, but other important criteria were also involved. Men or women who appeared to be informal leaders in their neighborhood, as well as the more formal and recognized community leaders, were selected for particular attention. By thus investing a little more in those who were leaders and those who seemed likely to be potentially influential, we expected that the rate of progress in the community as a whole would be increased.

Other reasons for visiting a particular home or group of homes were associated with action being taken at the time, or events such as the birth of a baby. A home may have decided to carry out a particular improvement, such as more intensive cultivation of its home vegetable garden, constructing a pit for the making of compost from refuse, or building a pit latrine; or a group of homes may have decided to protect the spring that was the source of their water supply. In all such cases, the community health worker would visit more often in order to maintain their interest and actively assist in the work.

The need for gathering data for periodic surveillance of family changes, seasonal changes in vegetable gardens, food storage, activities of different family members, dietary habit surveys, maintenance of housing and the environs of the home, and follow-through to families in need of social support at times of crises or changes were all important influences on the frequency with which homes were visited.

Group Discussions

The community health workers organized different groups in the community that came together to discuss their experiences and mutual problems, usually relevant to particular subjects or activities in which they were interested. The group once formed had a regular place and time of meeting. Trained in methods of organizing such groups, the community health workers were able to stimulate interest, introduce practical demonstrations and more authoritative talks when the groups wanted them, and help group members move from discussions to resolutions resulting in action by the members.

The discussion groups varied considerably in respect to their subject matter and membership, as well as in the ways they were initiated and developed. Many were organized as new groups for specific purposes, but often existing groups, such as a working party in the fields or a group of mothers attending the health center, were informally organized as a discussion group. Some groups were relatively short-lived, while others developed further, adding new members and continuing with their activities over long periods of time.

Some of the changes that occurred in a particular neighborhood indicate the results of the system of home visiting and group work. The neighborhood consisted of little more than 100 homes with a population of 750 people. Among the homes was that of a minister of the neighborhood church. He and his wife were well disposed toward the program of the health center, and the two community health workers in this area, a man and a woman, were well received in their home. It was not long before the woman community health worker organized a group of women, who met at this home and discussed a number of topics of interest to them, among which were the need for furthering school education and maternal and infant health. The male health worker and the minister followed this through in visits to the various homes of the neighborhood, meeting with the men of these homes. Eventually, this supportive action resulted in the community building a neighborhood primary school and maternal and child health subcenter, alongside one another. This subcenter was visited regularly by a family nurse and doctor, and the vast majority of mothers and babies in the area came to use it as a basic health service. A feature of this maternal and child health center was the group discussions of mothers, with community health worker and family nurse participation.

It is important to note that both community health workers in this area were born in Polela, received their primary education there, and then went elsewhere for further education before returning to their homes as teachers. Later they were recruited as community health educators, for which they had further special training at the Polela health center itself. Thus, men and women of this peasant community became important agents for the promotion of its health.

Utilization of Facilities at the
Health Center and Its Subcenters

The general clinic was a central feature of the health center. There was no restriction in its use, and patients attended from all parts of Polela itself, whether they lived in the health center's defined area or not. There were also many who lived considerable distances from the health center and would travel by foot or on horseback for several days, remaining with friends, kin, or special accommodations at the center while under treatment.

The clinic was an important screening instrument. Pregnant

women who attended were referred for their further care to special prenatal sessions. Infants were treated for their illnesses, and on recovery, discussions were held with their mothers and grandmothers, who were invited to bring their babies to the well-baby sessions at the health center. These were conducted by the same staff as the general clinic, with the family nurses having more responsibility for these sessions. Both the nurses and medical practitioners, physicians and medical aides, were thus responsible for preventive as well as curative work.

Expectant mothers and mothers with their babies and young children were encouraged to attend the health center for treatment of illness, as well as for health supervision through pregnancy, and for care of well babies. This was done in various ways, by community meetings especially with older women and men, with tribal chiefs and elders, and by visiting homes to discuss with families the facilities at the health center and the importance of their utilization.

Treatment of Sick Infants.   All families were invited to seek care at the health center as soon as a baby had signs of illness, or following accident or injury. The health education program emphasized:

1. Recognition of diarrhea before signs of dehydration appeared; the need to give urgent attention to the earliest signs of dehydration in infants with diarrhea; to attend for care at the health center even if using a traditional practitioner at the same time.
2. Recognition of signs of respiratory infection and the importance of early treatment.
3. Recognition of early signs of skin infections, and useful home treatments available from the health center.
4. Burns, snakebites, and other injuries. The immediate first aid measures were taught, and attendance at the health center as soon as possible was encouraged.

The treatment program by the health center included certain basic routines, which all members of the clinic staff could carry out. These were treatment of diarrhea and dehydration, acute bronchitis and pneumonia, burns, snakebite, and treatments for scabies and impetigo. Attention to nutritional status was an essential part of the care of all cases.

The number of babies brought to the health center was a striking feature of the response of the population to the care facilities which were developed. Over 80 percent of 0- to 2-year-olds in the population attended in the course of one of the early years, with no sex difference.

Prenatal Care

Prenatal care was one of the earliest services that was heavily utilized, and in the course of several years over 90 percent of mothers recorded as having given birth had used the health center for their prenatal care. Among the important routines were examinations of blood specimens for serologic tests for syphilis (Wasserman) and hemoglobin estimations. Low hemoglobin values were very rare, but positive Wasserman tests were common. Gonorrhea too was not uncommon. The treatment of syphilis and gonorrhea was a central feature of the program.

The outcome of pregnancy was markedly affected by the treatment of pregnant women with positive Wasserman reactions. Over a period of 5 successive years, during which the records of outcome of pregnancy were measured, there was a marked decline in the stillbirth rate of such mothers:

Births to Mothers Treated for Syphilis During Pregnancy

| | *Births* | *Stillbirths* | |
Year	*No.*	*No.*	*%*
1	60	9	15.0
2	68	7	10.3
3	77	4	5.2
4	66	5	7.5
5	54	1	1.9

Not only was this measurable effect of prenatal care important, but there was a marked decline in the incidence of new cases of syphilis, which is referred to later in this chapter.

Nutrition Work with Expectant Mothers. The poor nutritional state of expectant mothers was an important finding of our community diagnosis, and indicated the need for action. Their short stature was a product of a life of poverty and malnutrition, which only a long-term program for the promotion of child growth and nutrition might eventually modify. However, there was a case for action to improve the nutritional status of the women through pregnancy and lactation. The action taken was improvement of diet by dispensing milk powder, vitaminized oil (A and D), and other vitamin supplements. In those homes having cows in milk, the families were encouraged to use milk for expectant and lactating mothers, as well as for infants. Young married women, who by custom came to live in their husband's family home, were not permitted to drink the milk of its cows until they had been ceremonially received and accepted into the home. This involved us in a number of family discussions to hasten the necessary process for acceptance, thus permitting her use of milk.

The use of the products of home gardens was also examined, and dietary advice given on the basis of availability, at the same time as the health education program for improvement of home gardens was proceeding. Those women who were able attended the weekly educational gardening sessions held in the health center's large demonstration garden. They participated in the work, attended cookery demonstrations, and took home a supply of mixed vegetables.

Infant Nutrition and Weight Growth

Promotion of improved nutrition of infants and young children was a most important community health program. Not only was malnutrition a feature of many cases of illness, but it was a general condition determining failure of growth even in those classified as well babies.

The aims of the program were:

1. To gather data on infant feeding practices, the prevailing concepts of the role of feeding and nutrition in various illnesses, the foods available that might be used for improved feeding practices, and the potential for improving food resources.
2. The promotion of growth, especially weight growth.
3. Prevention of nutritional failure, such as kwashiorkor and marasmus.
4. Improved nutritional management of ill children.

Our approach was initially education of families in recognizing malnutrition and understanding the basis for modifying the diet accordingly. In doing this the focus of the program was on:

Breast Feeding. The early commencement of breast feeding. Encouragement of the customary practice in the community, namely, prolonged breast feeding and "adjusted" feeding as opposed to any fixed time schedule.

Other Foods. Gradual introduction of other foods, namely,

Milk and its products, with vitamin supplements.
Introduction of potatoes and pumpkins.
Mixed cereal feeding in place of maize only.

Dried legumes.
Green vegetables.
Eggs, poultry, meat.

Milk powders, full cream, and skim milk were available at the health center for issue at well-baby sessions, in addition to their use in treatment of sick children. Beans and cowpeas, which were commonly grown, were encouraged. Soya beans were grown in the demonstration garden at the health center, and suitable methods of preparation were shown to mothers. The seeds were then introduced to those homes expressing an interest in this legume.

A major problem was the predominance of a single cereal, maize, as a weaning food. The desirability of widening the variety of foods was clear. When the health center was first established, the main vegetables in the home gardens were maize, pumpkins, beans, and potatoes. Our surveys showed that potatoes and pumpkins were the most commonly grown vegetables in the summer gardens. A further study indicated that the women, mothers and grandmothers, would be willing to use these in the feeding of infants and young children if shown how to prepare suitable feeds. With some experimentation we prepared a potato-pumpkin-milk mixture, ranging from a thin gruel to a thicker mash. This slowly became popular, and with the addition of sorghum and legumes to the feeding of older infants and young children, the variety for which we aimed was introduced.

Vegetable Growing.   While the infant feeding program was being developed, the wider objective of improving home vegetable production for better feeding of all members of the family was actively pursued. We encouraged the home making of compost from refuse in the homes, gardens, poultry, and cattle enclosures, and its use in the home gardens. A seed-buying cooperative was started, and a market for exchange and sale of products was established at the health center by the people.

The involvement of the community in developing home gardening of vegetables was one of the most effective of the nutritional programs of the health center. Detailed seasonal surveys of vegetable growing in gardens were carried out by the health center over many years. There was an increase in the proportion of homes growing vegetables in the summer as well as winter seasons, and more varieties of vegetables were grown. Thus, while in the first year of the health center's establishment 76 percent of homes had vegetable gardens, the majority growing only two varieties, pumpkin and potatoes, within 3 years of the vegetable growing program this had increased to 21 varieties, and 10 years after its initiation 33 varieties were being grown. The proportion of homes with summer gardens in the rainy season was 89 percent, and in the dry winter 69 percent of homes were growing vegetables.

An important effect of this home gardening program was the wider variety of vegetables used in infant and child feeding. The community became very enthusiastic about the gardening program, and there was keen competition in increasing the amount and variety of vegetables produced.

Change in Weight Growth of Infants

Earlier in this chapter, we presented the weight growth of moderately well babies during the earlier years of the health center practice, and the criteria used in defining such infants were outlined. Summarizing the findings, weight growth was satisfactory during the first 3 to 4 months of age, after which there was increasing retardation.

It was thought that the infant feeding regime was the main explanation of the weight growth trend in those "well babies." The satisfactory growth in the earlier months was probably a direct result of the successful initiation and maintenance of an adjusted breast-feeding relationship. The increasing degree of retardation, from the middle months of the year through to the end of the first year, was considered by us to be due to failure to meet the needs for other foods in the weaning process. The limited amount of cows' milk available and its seasonal variation, the very limited use of eggs, meat, fresh vegetables, and the predominance of one cereal, maize, were clear evidence of the main inadequacies.

The changes advised by the health team, which it actively helped to encourage and make feasible, have been outlined. This, together with more effective treatment of illness and its primary prevention, is in our view the main reason for the changes shown in Figure 9-1, which is based on data of well babies' weights, gathered over a period of 5 to 10 years later, as far as possible using the same criteria.

It is evident that well babies, as so defined, were superior in weight after 10 years of the health center program in the community. The difference between the earlier and later weight curves was significant after the age of 5 months, and the superiority of the later cohort became more evident beyond this age. The changing community picture, as represented by these two weight curves, may be interpreted with other variables as an indicator of improved infant health. In par-

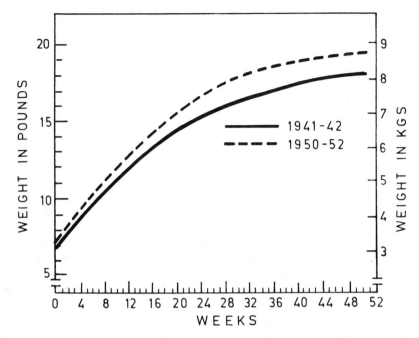

FIG. 9-1.   Change in weight growth of well babies in Polela 10 years after the establishment of a special health center program. [Adapted from Slome, 1962 (see Ref. 7).]

ticular, improved weight growth was associated with a marked decline in the infant mortality rates.

Kwashiorkor.   The failure in weight growth in the second half of the first year, which our early observations indicated, was probably the first sign of a subsequent condition of protein malnutrition. As the infant's demand for more food increased and the amount of breast milk declined to the point where the child was completely weaned to other foods, there were marked protein and vitamin deficiencies in the diet. It was at this time that some of the children developed the syndrome of kwashiorkor, which in Polela reached its peak incidence in the second year, following complete weaning from breast feeding to other foods. The diet and nutrition program outlined had an important impact on the incidence of kwashiorkor, which declined from 15 per 1000 children aged 0 to 2 years, over the 3-year period, 1948 to 1950, to 3 per 1000 of this age over the following 3 years, 1951 to 1953. Over the same periods, a similar decline in the incidence of kwashiorkor occurred in the children aged 3 to 5 years, from 6 to 3 per 1000.[7]

Later, an increase in incidence of kwashiorkor was observed. Whereas only 17 cases were reported in 1956, during the following 2 years 53 and 61 cases were known to have occurred. This was thought to be due to an increasing protein shortage. Despite this increased incidence of kwashiorkor, the case mortality rate decreased with effective treatment.[8]

While diet was the main determinant of kwashiorkor, there were factors influencing both the diet and breakdown in acute nutritional failure. These included communicable diseases, such as tuberculous infection, whooping cough, measles, and the common gastroenteritis. In all such illnesses, for successful therapy, it was vital to pay attention to the threat they posed to the nutritional status of the child. Hence, all medical therapy in such cases included dietary supplements. Similarly, special attention was given by the health center to deprived children. This included the displaced child who would be removed from the breast completely, as soon as the mother knew she was pregnant again, to children deprived of their mothers because of the latter's illness, or being left with grandmothers in Polela while their mothers were away in a city for work or visiting their husbands. This kind of knowledge was readily available, having been obtained by the community health workers in their close contact with the community and its families.

The Control and Treatment of Communicable Diseases

While much of our attention was focused on promotion of improved nutrition in infancy, an important concurrent problem, itself a cause of malnutrition, was the high incidence of a number of communicable diseases. The high prevalence rate of syphilis in expectant mothers in itself required that we encourage as many expectant mothers as possible to use the facilities of the health center. There was an encouraging response, allowing us to screen all cases and provide the most suitable treatment available at the time. Syphilis, tuberculosis, and other serious communicable diseases such as typhoid fever, whooping cough, and measles were common. The frequency of less specific diseases, gastroenteritis through the summer and acute upper respiratory infections, acute bronchitis, and pneumonia through the autumn to early spring, necessitated active health education for increased use of the health center by mothers with infants. Rehydration and feeding in gastroenteritis and treatment of pneumonia were important secondary prevention measures, which were readily appreciated by the community. Primary prevention of these conditions, especially gastroenteritis, was focused on nutrition and hygienic feeding habits, using clean utensils, with discouragement of bottle feeding because mothers did not have the facilities needed for clean bottles. Skin infections, scabies, and impetigo were readily treated and controlled by treatment of all members of the family at home.

Immunization included smallpox vaccination; tetanus, whooping cough, diphtheria (triple vaccine); typhoid-paratyphoid endotoxoid.

The doctors maintained charts of acute illness; these were reviewed daily and at the weekly staff conferences, which included the community health workers. Communicable diseases in infants were thus recorded and reviewed, with follow-through to their homes where necessary. The charts became a useful visual means of following the seasonal changes of acute illnesses.

Change in Environmental Determinants. There were active attempts to interest individual families and the community as a whole in changing the immediate hazards to health in their environment. When the health center was established, all homes were using water from springs, or sometimes streams and rivers, with no protection of the source from pollution; and no homes had constructed pit latrines or special pits for the composting of domestic, garden, and animal refuse. Appreciating the importance of compost for enriching their garden soil, within 10 years 43 percent of the homes in the defined area had compost pits in which they were disposing of refuse, but only 8 percent had constructed pit latrines. The reasons for resistance to the construction of pit latrines by each home was that these would facilitate access to feces, an intimate bodily substance, which the people believed might be used by ill-wishers to cause a person or family harm. Therefore, something was needed which would put excreta beyond the reach of such persons—for example, a water-borne disposal system that the people of Polela had seen in cities.

The health center's program for the protection of water supplies was more acceptable. It involved the construction of concrete reservoirs built into the hillside, enclosing the spring, with a tap and overflow pipe. The families sharing the spring would be involved in a number of discussions with the community health workers, and would themselves construct the reservoir with help from the health center team. Within 8 years of the start of this particular program, 26 percent of the homes in the defined area were using water from such protected springs.

Noteworthy Changes in the Incidence and Prevalence of Some Communicable Diseases. Soon after the initiation of the health center we were called upon to investigate and control a number of epidemics of serious diseases, namely, typhoid and typhus fevers and smallpox. Within a 12-month period, there were no less than five confirmed outbreaks of typhoid fever. Several of these were in neighborhoods that were later included by the health center in its defined area of action. In one outbreak, by the time we were called in, deaths had already occurred in 27 homes, 19 percent of all the homes in the affected area, and of the 46 persons who had died only 12 had attended a physician. Modern concepts of causation were unknown. With the development of our community-oriented primary care program, such epidemics ceased in the defined area, but the health center team was still requested to control epidemics in parts beyond the defined area of the health center. We related this striking change to several factors, namely, the environmental health program, the extensive immunizations and vaccinations, and early recognition of the cases that occurred.

Less dramatic, but nevertheless important, was the decline in incidence of whooping cough, and in the mortality from this disease, and measles. The former we considered to be a result of immunization, and the latter of improved nutrition in infants and the treatment given to cases. There was also a marked decline in scabies and impetigo. The prevalence of infected patients attending the health center decreased from 17 to 2 percent over the 15-year period. These skin conditions were very much milder than previously, and when compared with cases from outside the defined area.

Syphilis. We have previously referred to the effects of treatment of syphilis in pregnancy. There was also a marked change in the incidence of new cases of the disease in the defined area, as illustrated by the following data: Over a 15-year period, 1942 to 1957, the incidence declined from 13.5 per 1000 population in our first year of measurement, through 6.7 in the third, 4.4 in the fifth, 1.5 in the tenth, and finally to 0.8 per 1000 in the fifteenth year. This was despite the widening defined area, with the consequent increase in population at risk, from less than 1000 in the first year, to over 5000 in the third, 6500 in the fifth, 8500 in the tenth and 10,500 in the fifteenth.

We related this change to the intensive education of the community about the disease and its transmission, the need for periodic examinations, and our intensive case-finding program followed by treatment. In the earlier years, treatment was by use of arsenicals, and later by penicillin.

Similar progress was reported for gonorrhea; the rate of new diagnosed cases decreased from 17 in 1951 to 2 per 1000 of the total population in the defined area in 1957.

Tuberculosis. This disease was the single most important cause of death in the adult population, and contributed significantly to morbidity and mortality in infants and young children. The routine examination of babies and young children included periodic tuberculin testing, a measure that allowed for early diagnosis of infection in the individual child and the family. We were not able to effect any appreciable change in the incidence of infection, nor in the morbidity and mortality caused by the disease. In one area studied through a year, 8 percent of the homes had at least one member known to have tuberculosis, and these homes constituted 30 percent of the total homes in which a death had occurred during that year.

We considered that the continued seriousness of the disease, and the high incidence of infection, were related to several factors that we were not able to influence at the time. The infection was often introduced to the home by tuberculotic men returning sick from the city, when they were unable to continue working. When children became infected and sick, the family did not asssociate their illness with that of the sick man, whose sickness was diagnosed as a traditional syndrome of "poisoning of the chest," caused by an ill-wisher. Added to this was the poor nutritional status of the majority of people, which made them more susceptible to the disease.

THE CHANGING INFANT MORTALITY RATE (IMR)

The introduction of a system of demographic surveillance, which included the recording of all births and deaths, allowed for calculation of infant mortality rates. Comparing four periods of time over a 15-year period, there was a decline in the IMR from 25.3 percent of live births during the first 2-year period, to 8.6 percent in the last 2-year period (Table 9-4). While this change is suggestive of the health center's influence, it is not in itself an evaluation of the health center's program.

In order to evaluate the infant health program, we carried out an analysis of the records of five areas during the first year in which the particular area of homes was incorporated into the community-oriented primary health care service (Table 9-5). By combining the findings in the "new" areas included during the period 1942 to 1944, and comparing them with those added some years later, 1950 and 1951, there was a difference in the IMR, 25.6 percent and 18.9 percent.

TABLE 9-4

Infant Mortality Rates in Four Periods
Between 1942 and 1956[8,9]

2-YEAR PERIODS	LIVE BIRTHS RECORDED	DEATHS UNDER 1 YEAR	IMR (%)
1942–1943	150	38	25.3
1945–1946	490	89	18.2
1950–1951	637	68	10.7
1955–1956	720	62	8.6

This was not found to be significant, and thus we combined them as a control group for purposes of comparison with the families who had been in the community-oriented primary care program for longer than 1 year.

Infant Mortality Rate in "Old" and "New" Defined Areas

A comparison of the IMR in the new areas with those incorporated in the community-oriented primary care service for a longer period showed that the total IMR in the control areas, that is, the five areas shown in Table 9-5, during the first year of their incorporation in the defined area, was 24.2 percent. The corresponding figures for the old areas (intervention group) in these same years were 82 infant deaths of 729 live births, an IMR of 11.2 percent. The difference between the

TABLE 9-5

Infant Mortality Found During the First Year
in Which a Particular Group of Families Was Incorporated
in the Defined Area Service[9]

NEW AREA	NUMBER OF LIVE BIRTHS	NUMBER OF INFANT DEATHS	IMR (%)
1942	40	11	27.5 ⎫
1943	81	23	28.4 ⎬ 25.6
1944	78	17	21.8 ⎭
1950	19	4	21.1 ⎫ 18.9
1951	34	6	17.7 ⎭
Total of 5 areas during their first year in the defined area	252	61	24.2

control and intervention groups was not only large, but highly significant.

The superiority of the intervention group, which has been demonstrated, was already becoming apparent in the first 3 years of the program. The IMR in the new families, added in each of the years 1942, 1943, and 1944, was 25.6 percent, whereas in the old families that were in their second or third year in the program, in the years 1942 and 1943, it had already dropped to 16.6 percent.

The major differences between the old and the new areas were in the kinds of service provided. All families, whether included in the defined area or not, had access to the services at the health center itself. It must be remembered that these included preventive and curative services. The outstanding difference between the two groups was in the services provided by the community health workers in the homes and their immediate neighborhoods in the community. This was an integral part of the community-oriented primary care provided to the families in the defined area of homes, and not provided to the areas that had not yet been incorporated. In the latter areas, the homes were only visited in exceptional circumstances, such as when the health center intervened to help control an epidemic, or when there was a serious case needing attention.

The field health education was, as indicated earlier, closely integrated with the services provided to these families at the health center itself. It seemed to us then, and even more so now on looking back, that the differences between the two kinds of service were not the technical aspects of diagnosis and treatment, nor accessibility to the health center's clinics, but rather the nature of the relationship developed between the health center team and the community. This was a result of the intensive and informal health education program, which took community health workers into the homes and neighborhoods of the defined area. It was in this way that the emphasis of the service was modified from what is usually done for patients to what the family or community does for itself, assisted by the health center team.

REFERENCES*

1. McCarrison R: Studies in Deficiency Disease. London, Oxford Medical Publications, 1921

*For more details on the Polela Health Centre, see References 5 to 17 of Chapter 8.

2. Kark SL: Nutrition and Adjustment in the Changing Society of Polela. Doctoral thesis, Univ. Witwatersrand Library, 1953

3. Omran AR, Standley CC: Family Formation Patterns and Health. Geneva, WHO, 1976

4. Kark SL: The height and weight of men and women in relation to age, In Kark SL, Steuart GW (eds): A Practice of Social Medicine. Edinburgh, Livingstone, 1962, p 186

5. ———: A community syndrome of malnutrition, communicable diseases and mental-ill health in a rural community. In Epidemiology and Community Medicine. New York, Appleton, 1974, p 269

6. ———: The social pathology of syphilis in Africans. S Afr Med J 23:77, 1949

7. Slome C: Community health in rural Polela. In Kark SL, Steuart GW (eds): A Practice of Social Medicine. Edinburgh, Livingstone, 1962, p 280

8. Bennett FJ: Mortality in a rural Zulu community. Br J Prev Soc Med 14:1, 1960

9. Kark SL, Cassel J: The Polela Health Centre. S Afr Med J 26:101, 131, 1952

INDEX

Italic letters following page numbers indicate tables or figures.